# Dealing with the Menopause

CRAFTED BY SKRIUWER

Copyright © 2024 by Skriuwer.

All rights reserved. No part of this book may be used or reproduced in any form whatsoever without written permission except in the case of brief quotations in critical articles or reviews.

For more information, contact : **kontakt@skriuwer.com** (www.skriuwer.com)

# TABLE OF CONTENTS

## CHAPTER 1: INTRODUCTION TO MENOPAUSE

- What menopause is and why it occurs
- Typical age range and variations
- Early or late menopause considerations
- Overall importance of understanding menopause

## CHAPTER 2: MENOPAUSE BASICS—HORMONES AND STAGES

- Perimenopause, menopause, and post-menopause timeline
- Key hormonal shifts in estrogen and progesterone
- How these stages affect the body and mind

## CHAPTER 3: KEY HORMONES—HOW THEY AFFECT THE BODY

- Role of estrogen, progesterone, and other hormones
- Influences on bone, mood, and metabolism
- Signs of hormone imbalances

## CHAPTER 4: MAJOR BODY CHANGES DURING MENOPAUSE

- Internal system adjustments (reproductive, circulatory, etc.)
- Physical and mental shifts tied to hormone drops
- How these changes vary among women

## CHAPTER 5: PHYSICAL SHIFTS & HOW TO MANAGE THEM

- Hot flashes, night sweats, and body temperature swings
- Muscle aches or stiffness and practical remedies
- Techniques for daily comfort (clothing, room adjustments)

## CHAPTER 6: EMOTIONAL CHANGES AND BALANCE

- Reasons for mood swings, irritability, or sadness
- Simple methods to calm the mind
- Discussing emotional needs with loved ones

## CHAPTER 7: SLEEP CONCERNS AND ENERGY LEVELS

- *Common sleep problems in menopause (insomnia, restlessness)*
- *Routine changes that support deeper rest*
- *Daytime tips to boost energy and alertness*

## CHAPTER 8: WEIGHT AND BODY SHAPE CHANGES

- *Why extra pounds often appear around the waist*
- *Balancing diet, metabolism, and physical activity*
- *Managing healthy weight without extreme dieting*

## CHAPTER 9: BONE HEALTH AND STRENGTH

- *Risk of osteoporosis and bone thinning*
- *Importance of calcium, vitamin D, and weight-bearing exercise*
- *Practical steps to protect and build strong bones*

## CHAPTER 10: SEXUAL HEALTH AND INTIMACY

- *How dryness and hormonal shifts affect closeness*
- *Open communication with partners*
- *Options for increasing comfort and confidence*

## CHAPTER 11: HEART HEALTH AND CIRCULATION

- *Why heart concerns can rise after menopause*
- *Keeping blood pressure and cholesterol in check*
- *Daily habits that benefit the heart and blood vessels*

## CHAPTER 12: SKIN AND HAIR CHANGES

- *Dryness, wrinkles, and hair thinning causes*
- *Gentle skincare and hair care routines*
- *Practical tips for boosting comfort and appearance*

## CHAPTER 13: NUTRITION AND MEAL PLANNING

- *Key nutrients for menopausal and post-menopausal bodies*
- *Balancing proteins, healthy fats, and fiber*
- *Meal ideas and food prep strategies*

## CHAPTER 14: PHYSICAL ACTIVITY AND MOVEMENT

- *Importance of regular exercise for bone, muscle, and mood*
- *Types of exercise (cardio, strength, flexibility)*
- *Simple routines to fit different lifestyles*

## CHAPTER 15: EVALUATING HORMONE THERAPIES

- *How hormone treatments work and who they help*
- *Benefits vs. possible risks*
- *Speaking with a doctor to make safe decisions*

## CHAPTER 16: NON-MEDICAL WAYS TO FEEL BETTER

- *Lifestyle shifts, herbal options, and relaxation*
- *Self-care ideas for hot flashes and dryness*
- *Everyday approaches for calmer moods*

## CHAPTER 17: MOOD CHANGES AND MENTAL HEALTH

- *Hormonal influences on emotions*
- *Recognizing deeper mood problems*
- *Strategies for emotional support and resilience*

## CHAPTER 18: HANDLING STRESS AT HOME AND WORK

- *Why stress can intensify during menopause*
- *Tools for organizing tasks and setting boundaries*
- *Quick calm-down methods and communication tips*

## CHAPTER 19: STAYING HEALTHY IN THE LONG TERM

- *Post-menopause outlook on bone, heart, and mental health*
- *Screenings and checkups for ongoing well-being*
- *Balancing lifestyle habits for years ahead*

## CHAPTER 20: PRACTICAL STEPS FOR DAILY LIFE

- *Making consistent routines for nutrition and exercise*
- *Managing stress, rest, and social connections*
- *Building a flexible plan that adapts as needs change*

# Chapter 1: Introduction to Menopause

Menopause is a natural change that happens in a woman's life as she grows older. Even though it is natural, many people do not talk about it openly. This can lead to confusion and fear, because there is not enough clear information that is easy to understand. Menopause often brings changes in the body and mind that can make a woman feel worried or uneasy. Knowing more about it can help a woman feel better prepared and more at peace when facing these shifts.

In this chapter, we will discuss what menopause is, how people have understood it over time, and why it matters to learn about it today. We will also look at the average age at which women go through menopause and why some women may reach it earlier or later than others. Finally, we will talk about the value of knowing what happens during menopause, so that women can make smart choices about their health, daily activities, and personal comfort.

## What is Menopause?

Menopause is marked by a point in time when a woman no longer has menstrual periods. Usually, doctors say that a woman has gone through menopause if she has not had a period for 12 months in a row. This change happens because the ovaries stop releasing eggs on a regular schedule. At the same time, the ovaries slow down the release of certain hormones that are linked to the menstrual cycle.

Though it marks the end of monthly cycles, menopause also involves other changes in the body. Some women notice changes in their mood, their energy, and even in how they handle daily tasks. Each woman may have a different set of signs, and these can vary in severity. There is no single way that everyone goes through menopause, because each woman's body is special in its own way.

## Age and Timing

The average age for menopause is usually around 51 years old, but there is a wide range for what is considered normal. Some women may notice signs in their mid-40s, while others may not have clear signs until their late 50s. The word "signs" here refers to things like hot flashes, missed periods, or changes in mood. Some women reach menopause early due to health conditions, medical treatments, or hereditary factors. Early menopause can happen before age 40, which is called premature menopause. Some women experience menopause closer to age 45, which is sometimes called early menopause.

Late menopause usually refers to women who do not reach menopause until around 55 or older. This may be linked to family history or certain health factors. Regardless of whether menopause happens early, late, or at the average age, it is important for each woman to be aware of the changes happening in her body. Understanding these changes can help her make sense of mood swings, changes in weight, or other shifts that might otherwise cause stress.

## Social and Cultural Views

Over the years, different cultures have had different beliefs and attitudes about menopause. In some places, people did not talk much about it. In other places, there have been various ideas about why menopause happens and what it means. For example, in some parts of the world, older women are given respect because of their age and wisdom, and menopause is simply seen as a stage of growing older. In other communities, there may be less open discussion. In these settings, women might not feel comfortable asking questions or seeking help for changes they notice.

In modern times, there is more talk about menopause in health magazines, online forums, and at doctor's offices. However, there is still confusion and wrong information spread in some places. Some people think that menopause signals the end of a woman's ability to be active or healthy, which is not true. Many women stay healthy and active for decades after menopause. Clear and factual information can help correct these misunderstandings and ease any concerns.

## Why Knowledge Matters

It is often said that knowledge can help reduce fear. This is especially true when it comes to changes in the body. Menopause can bring many new experiences, but if a woman knows why they are happening and what she can do, she is more likely to feel calm. Without this information, she may feel lost or think that something is wrong with her. For instance, if she is unaware that the drop in certain hormones can affect her mood, she might blame herself for feeling irritable.

When a woman understands the reasons behind changes, she can seek solutions that work for her. That might mean talking to her doctor, trying certain foods, or adjusting her daily routine. The key is to have enough accurate information to make healthy choices. A woman who is well-informed might also be more open to speaking about her worries with her friends or family members. This can create a support network and reduce stress.

## Personal Stories as Helpful Examples

Some women find it helpful to hear stories from others who have already experienced menopause. While these are not medical advice, they can offer real-life insights. Hearing how another woman handled hot flashes at work, for example, might give new ideas for staying cool and confident. Some women learn about adding more calcium to their meals to support bone health by talking to friends who have done so. These stories can guide a woman through her own process.

It is important to remember, though, that each woman's body is different. What works for one person might not be helpful for another. Still, there can be comfort in knowing that others have faced similar concerns. Gathering many points of view can help a woman find the mix of tools that help her the most.

## Body Changes: An Overview

Menopause involves many shifts that may affect both the body and the mind. A quick preview might include:

- **Hot flashes**: Sudden bursts of warmth, often in the upper body and face.
- **Night sweats**: Hot flashes that happen during sleep, which may lead to waking up sweaty.

- **Irregular periods**: Changes in the length or heaviness of menstrual cycles, eventually ending.
- **Changes in mood**: Feelings of sadness, anxiety, or irritability may increase.
- **Physical changes**: Some women notice changes in how their body stores fat.

We will talk about these topics in much more detail in later chapters. For now, it is enough to know that menopause can affect many areas of daily life.

---

## The Importance of Discussing Menopause

Menopause is a major change for many women. It does not only affect her body, but also her emotions, relationships, and daily comfort. When women do not talk about it, they may miss helpful tips or words of advice. They might also feel alone in their experiences, which can make any physical or emotional discomfort feel worse.

Open discussion can lead to more support, whether from friends, health experts, or community groups. It is also useful for younger women to learn about menopause ahead of time, so they can be ready when it happens to them. Some may be caring for older family members and want to understand what they might be going through. It is good for everyone to have correct information, so that menopause is not seen as a scary or shameful topic.

---

## The Role of Doctors and Health Professionals

Health professionals, such as general doctors, women's health doctors (gynecologists), and even mental health experts, can be very helpful during menopause. They can answer questions, do tests to check hormone levels, and suggest treatments if needed. Some might refer a woman to nutrition experts, physical therapists, or counselors, depending on her specific concerns. It is wise for a woman to have regular check-ups during this time to monitor her overall health. Blood pressure, weight, and bone density are examples of measurements that might need to be watched.

Women who have existing health problems, such as diabetes or high blood pressure, should be sure to talk with their doctors about how menopause might affect these conditions. Sometimes, small changes in medication or diet can help keep everything on track.

## Shattering Myths

There are many myths about menopause. Here are a few examples:

1. **Myth**: Menopause is the same for everyone.
   **Reality**: Each woman's body responds in its own way. The kinds of signs and their strength can vary a lot.
2. **Myth**: Menopause always causes big mood swings.
   **Reality**: While changes in hormones can affect mood, not everyone has large mood swings.
3. **Myth**: Menopause ends a woman's active life.
   **Reality**: Menopause is a phase, not an end. Many women stay active, enjoy activities, and do everything they used to do.
4. **Myth**: Menopause is only about hot flashes.
   **Reality**: It can affect many areas, including bones, heart health, and mental well-being.

Knowing the facts can help a woman avoid believing these myths. When people spread wrong ideas, it can add to stress or confusion. By reading trustworthy sources and talking to health experts, women can get the correct information.

## The Emotional Side of Menopause

While the body goes through changes, emotions can also shift. Some women talk about feeling a sense of sadness because they can no longer have children, even if they did not plan to have any more. Others feel relieved to be free from monthly periods or the worry of getting pregnant. Some feel anxious about how their bodies are changing.

All these feelings can be valid. It is normal to have mixed emotions about a life change that affects so many things. That is why finding healthy ways to talk about or handle these emotions is key. This might include talking to friends, meeting with a counselor, or keeping track of feelings in a journal. These steps can help reduce stress and make the transition smoother.

## Lifestyle Factors That Affect Menopause

The way a woman lives can influence how she feels during menopause. Factors such as diet, exercise habits, and stress levels play a role. For instance, a woman who eats balanced meals with enough calcium and vitamin D may find it easier to maintain bone strength. A woman who exercises a few times a week might notice that she sleeps better or feels less stressed.

Smoking is another factor that can make menopause more difficult. Research shows that women who smoke often reach menopause earlier and may have worse hot flashes. Cutting down on smoking or quitting entirely can help. Alcohol use can also influence how a woman feels during menopause. While some women might enjoy a small glass of wine, drinking too much can add to sleep problems or mood changes.

## Menopause and Family Life

Menopause can affect relationships with a spouse, children, or even extended family. Mood changes may make a woman feel less patient. Physical discomforts like night sweats could cause poor sleep, which might lead to more irritability during the day. Loved ones may not always understand what she is going through, especially if there is little discussion about it.

Having calm and open talks with family members can be helpful. A partner might appreciate knowing why a woman wakes up at night or why she may not feel as interested in certain activities. A daughter or son might want to learn about these changes so they can offer support or simply understand what is happening. Clear communication can lower tension at home and help everyone adjust.

## Looking Ahead

Menopause is not a simple event that happens overnight. It is a process that can last for several years. There is a stage called perimenopause that happens before menopause, where hormonal changes begin. Menopause itself is the point at which 12 months pass without a period. After that, a woman is in post-menopause. We will talk about these stages in the next chapter.

The key idea here is that menopause is not something to fear. It is a natural change, and with the right information, a woman can handle it in a way that fits her life. She can take steps to stay healthy, seek medical support if needed, and talk about any emotional or mental concerns with trusted people.

---

## Summary of Chapter 1

In this first chapter, we looked at what menopause is and why it matters to talk about it. We learned that menopause is the point when a woman no longer has menstrual periods, usually confirmed after 12 months without a period. The average age is around 51, but it varies from woman to woman. Some may reach it earlier, while others later. We also discussed how cultural views of menopause can differ, and how myths can spread confusion.

We talked about the importance of knowing the facts, because it helps reduce worries. We noted some common signs, like hot flashes and mood changes, but these do not affect every woman in the same way. We spoke about the need to maintain a healthy lifestyle and have open communication with loved ones to handle menopause more smoothly.

From here, we will move on to a more detailed look at what happens inside the body during menopause, focusing on hormones and the stages (perimenopause, menopause, and post-menopause). Understanding the science behind menopause can help explain why some of the changes happen, and it may help women make more informed choices about their health.

---

# Chapter 2: Menopause Basics: Hormones and Stages

In the previous chapter, we introduced menopause as the time when a woman's menstrual periods stop permanently. We also discussed common myths and reasons why clear information is so valuable. This chapter focuses on the basics of how menopause unfolds, with a spotlight on key hormones. We will also learn about the different stages: perimenopause, menopause, and post-menopause. Each stage brings its own patterns of hormonal shifts that can impact a woman's daily life.

The body's chemistry is at the core of menopause. Hormones are chemical messengers that tell the body what to do. In this phase of a woman's life, some of these hormones rise or fall in different ways than before. By knowing what is happening inside the body, women can better understand the signs they may notice. This chapter will explore how hormones like estrogen and progesterone operate and why the body changes in the ways it does.

## What Are Hormones?

Hormones are substances that travel through the bloodstream to tissues and organs. They help control many processes, such as growth, metabolism, mood, and reproduction. During a woman's reproductive years, certain hormones work together to regulate the monthly cycle. For example, the body releases estrogen and progesterone to prepare for a possible pregnancy. If no pregnancy happens, the body sheds the lining of the uterus, and this becomes the menstrual flow.

As a woman approaches menopause, her ovaries begin to release less of these hormones. At times, the levels may even fluctuate widely, going up and down in a seemingly unpredictable way. This fluctuation can lead to hot flashes, mood swings, and changes in monthly cycles. Understanding these hormone shifts is key to making sense of the physical and emotional changes that often come with menopause.

# Key Hormones in Menopause

## Estrogen

Estrogen is one of the main hormones involved in female development and reproductive health. It helps manage the menstrual cycle and also contributes to bone strength, heart health, and more. When menopause is near, the ovaries slow down the production of estrogen, causing the overall levels to drop. This dip in estrogen is the reason for many of the shifts in the body. For instance, low estrogen can lead to dryness in certain parts of the body and can affect how the skin feels.

## Progesterone

Progesterone works closely with estrogen to support the menstrual cycle. It helps prepare the uterus for pregnancy after ovulation. When menopause approaches, progesterone levels also change. During the perimenopause stage, the production of progesterone can become inconsistent. Some months, the body may produce more, and other months less. This can affect the regularity and heaviness of menstrual periods.

## Follicle-Stimulating Hormone (FSH)

The brain releases a hormone called FSH to signal the ovaries to mature eggs. As a woman ages, and her ovaries become less active, the brain tries harder to stimulate them, so it releases more FSH. Doctors often measure FSH levels in a blood test to check for signs of menopause. Higher levels of FSH are a sign that the body is responding to lower hormone output from the ovaries.

## Luteinizing Hormone (LH)

LH is another hormone that helps manage the menstrual cycle. Like FSH, it also comes from the brain. It helps with ovulation and the release of eggs. During perimenopause, LH levels may go up and down. High levels of LH can combine with high FSH levels, giving doctors a signal that menopause is approaching.

# Perimenopause: The First Stage

Perimenopause is the stage leading up to menopause. It can start several years before the final menstrual period. Some women begin noticing changes in their 40s, but it can start earlier or later. During perimenopause, hormone levels, especially estrogen, can fluctuate a lot. This can cause some months to feel somewhat normal and others to bring strong hot flashes or other signs.

## Common Signs in Perimenopause

1. **Irregular Periods**: Some women may skip a few months, then have a very heavy flow, or have shorter cycles.
2. **Mood Changes**: Women may notice they are more irritable or feel down more often.
3. **Hot Flashes**: Periods of sudden warmth that often start in the chest and move upward.
4. **Sleep Problems**: Feeling restless at night or waking up sweating.

These signs can come and go. A woman might have them for a short time, then go for weeks or months with fewer issues. Over time, though, the ovaries produce less estrogen, and the body moves closer to menopause.

## Length of Perimenopause

The length of perimenopause can vary. For some women, it lasts just a few years, while others may notice changes for a decade. Since the signs can be inconsistent, it might be hard to know exactly when perimenopause starts. Doctors might use blood tests to look at hormone levels, but these tests can also show mixed results, because hormones can shift from day to day.

## Managing Perimenopause

Some women choose to talk with their doctors about how to handle the signs of perimenopause, especially if they are intense. Options may include birth control pills to help regulate cycles, or lifestyle changes like adjusting diet and exercise routines. Reducing stress can also be important, as stress can make some signs feel worse. Getting enough rest and seeking support from friends or family can be a big help during this stage.

# Menopause: The Official Mark

A woman is considered to have reached menopause once she has gone without a menstrual period for 12 months in a row. This is the official point that marks the end of her reproductive years. By this time, the ovaries are releasing very little estrogen, and eggs are no longer being prepared for fertilization in a predictable pattern. The average age at which women reach this point is around 51, but it can happen earlier or later.

## Confirming Menopause

Some women know they have reached menopause simply because their periods have completely stopped for a full year. Others might talk with a doctor and get blood tests to measure FSH levels. If the FSH levels are high, it is often a sign that the ovaries are not producing as much estrogen. This test, along with a review of signs, can confirm that menopause has occurred.

## Feelings at Menopause

Reaching menopause can stir up different feelings in different women. Some may feel relief from not having to deal with monthly cycles. Others may feel sad because it is tied to the end of fertility. There is no right or wrong way to feel. Often, emotions at menopause may be influenced by cultural ideas, personal beliefs, or family attitudes. Talking to a counselor or someone who understands can help if a woman feels overwhelmed.

---

# Post-Menopause: Life After the Final Period

Post-menopause starts after the 12-month mark without a period has been reached. During this time, signs like hot flashes may still continue, especially early on. However, for many women, the signs start to lessen in intensity. Each woman's experience is unique. Some may have hot flashes for a long time, while others see them fade quickly.

## Health Considerations After Menopause

Once in post-menopause, a woman's body produces much less estrogen. Low estrogen levels can affect various parts of the body, so it is often wise to pay special attention to long-term health. For example, bone density might decrease, so doctors often suggest calcium and vitamin D intake, along with regular weight-bearing exercise. Heart health becomes a bigger focus, as lower estrogen may raise certain risks. Regular check-ups can help identify any issues early.

**Emotional Well-Being**

Emotions can stabilize in post-menopause, but some women may still feel concerned about aging or changes in their bodies. Building a supportive circle of friends and family, or connecting with women who have similar experiences, can be helpful. Relaxation activities or counseling can also be good for dealing with worries. Each woman can find her own path to feeling balanced and confident during these years.

# How Long Does the Whole Process Take?

Menopause is not a single event but rather a series of changes that can stretch out over several years. Here is a rough outline of how long each phase might last:

- **Perimenopause**: Can start up to 10 years before menopause, but often lasts about 4 to 6 years.
- **Menopause**: Officially happens when a woman goes 12 months without a period.
- **Post-Menopause**: The years after menopause, which continue throughout the rest of a woman's life.

Some women move through these stages more quickly, while others may notice changes for a longer period. It is not always possible to predict exactly how long it will last for each individual.

# Early and Late Menopause

A small group of women go through menopause before 40. This is known as premature menopause. Reasons can include genetic factors, autoimmune diseases, or medical treatments like removing the ovaries or receiving cancer treatments. Women who experience early menopause may have a higher risk for bone loss and other issues because they spend more years with low estrogen levels. It is important for them to work closely with their doctors to protect their overall health.

Late menopause happens when a woman does not reach menopause until around 55 or older. Some might see late menopause as beneficial, because the body remains under the influence of estrogen for a longer time. However, doctors keep an eye on any related health risks, because late menopause can sometimes increase the likelihood of certain conditions, depending on family history or other factors.

## Common Questions About Hormones and Menopause

1. **Do all hormone levels drop at once?**
   Not exactly. Estrogen, progesterone, and other hormones may rise or fall in uneven patterns, especially during perimenopause. By the time menopause is reached, levels of estrogen and progesterone are generally much lower than before.
2. **What role do genetics play?**
   Genetics can influence when a woman starts perimenopause, how severe her signs might be, and how long the process lasts. If a woman's close relatives reached menopause early, she might also. However, lifestyle factors, diet, and overall health play a part too.
3. **Can stress affect hormone levels?**
   Stress can change how the brain and adrenal glands release certain hormones. While it may not directly cause menopause to start earlier, stress can affect how a woman feels and copes with the signs.
4. **How do doctors test for menopause?**
   Doctors sometimes use blood tests to check levels of FSH, LH, and estrogen. They also look at a woman's medical history and her signs. However, a single blood test might not be enough, since hormone levels can vary from day to day.

# Menopause vs. Other Hormonal Changes

Some women confuse the signs of menopause with other conditions that affect hormones. For example, thyroid problems can also cause mood swings or changes in energy. Polycystic Ovary Syndrome (PCOS) can make menstrual cycles irregular. If a woman is unsure if her signs are due to menopause, she should see a health professional who can run tests and rule out other possible causes. This helps ensure that she gets the correct guidance and care.

---

# Tips for Handling Hormone-Related Changes

1. **Track Your Cycles**: Keeping a journal of your menstrual periods can help you notice patterns in timing and flow. This is useful information to share with a doctor.
2. **Note Your Signs**: Write down when you have hot flashes, mood changes, or other issues. This can help identify what might trigger them, like certain foods or stress.
3. **Maintain a Balanced Diet**: Nutrient-rich foods give your body the building blocks it needs for healthy hormone function.
4. **Stay Active**: Gentle exercise like walking, yoga-like stretching (without using words you asked to avoid), or swimming can help keep your body strong and may balance hormones to some degree.
5. **Talk to a Doctor**: If signs become too hard to handle, it might be worth discussing hormone therapy or other treatment options.

---

# When to Seek Help

It is wise to see a doctor if any signs are making daily life very difficult, such as severe hot flashes that disturb sleep every night, or mood swings that cause strain in relationships. Extreme bleeding between periods or very heavy periods can also signal other issues. A doctor or health professional can conduct tests, provide advice, and suggest treatments if needed.

It is also important to note that hormone-related changes can affect mental well-being. Feelings of persistent sadness, worry, or a loss of interest in activities may need attention from a mental health expert. Sometimes, talking to a therapist or counselor can make a big difference. Proper medical support can help a woman handle menopause in a healthy, balanced manner.

## Overlap with Other Life Events

Many women experience menopause at a time in life when other major events are happening. Some are raising teenage children, while others may be caring for aging parents. Some might be at the height of their careers or thinking about retirement. These overlapping responsibilities and stressors can add to the difficulty. Knowing the stages of menopause and having a plan can make it easier to handle all these things without feeling lost.

## Preparing for the Next Chapters

Now that we have explored the basic stages of menopause and the main hormones involved, we can start to look at specific changes that happen in the body and mind. The next chapters will go into detail about things like major body changes, physical and emotional shifts, sleep problems, changes in weight, and more. By understanding the basic map of menopause, a woman can better grasp why these changes happen and what she can do about them.

Future chapters will also offer tips on how to handle these changes using simple methods at home, as well as information on talking with health professionals. The goal is to give a clear, in-depth look at what happens during menopause, so every woman can feel prepared to handle it in ways that make sense for her.

## Summary of Chapter 2

This chapter explained the three main stages of menopause: perimenopause, menopause, and post-menopause. We looked at the key hormones—estrogen, progesterone, FSH, and LH—and how they shift during each stage. Perimenopause is the lead-up phase when the ovaries start to produce less estrogen, and periods become irregular. Menopause is the point when a woman has gone 12 months without a period. Post-menopause follows and can continue for the rest of a woman's life, usually with very low hormone levels.

We discussed how a woman can confirm menopause, and why it is important to manage health concerns during and after the transition. We also covered some common questions about hormones and the effect of genetics. Finally, we provided some tips on keeping track of signs and seeking help when needed.

With this overview in mind, we will shift to more specific topics in the next chapters, such as physical shifts, emotional changes, and other detailed matters related to menopause.

# Chapter 3: Key Hormones—How They Affect the Body

In the first two chapters, we discussed the general idea of menopause, the basic timing of the stages, and the main hormones involved. Now, we will look more deeply at the ways these hormones work throughout the body. Menopause leads to changes in many systems, and these changes mostly tie back to the shifts in hormone levels. Understanding how these hormones interact with various tissues and organs can help a woman make better decisions for her well-being.

This chapter focuses on hormones that are most closely linked to menopause. We will look at how they help with key tasks like bone maintenance, blood flow, metabolism, and more. This includes hormones like estrogen, progesterone, and others that may not get as much attention but still play an important part in what a woman feels and observes during menopause. We will also touch on how different parts of the body—such as the brain, muscles, and immune system—can respond when hormone levels fall or shift.

---

## Estrogen Beyond the Menstrual Cycle

Many people think of estrogen only in terms of menstrual periods and fertility. In reality, estrogen has many other roles in the body. Before menopause, the ovaries are the main source of estrogen. After menopause, the ovaries slow or stop making it, and only small amounts come from other sources like fat tissue. These lower levels can affect many body processes.

### Bone Health and Estrogen

Estrogen helps protect bones by slowing the rate at which they lose minerals. Bones naturally break down and rebuild through a normal cycle. With enough estrogen, bones stay stronger because the balance of this cycle is controlled. Once estrogen levels drop, bone breakdown may happen faster than bone rebuilding. This can raise the chance of thinning bones. This is why many experts suggest checking bone health during or after menopause.

**Estrogen and Body Temperature**

One common sign of menopause is hot flashes. These happen because the body's temperature controls become more sensitive as estrogen drops. Parts of the brain that handle temperature regulation can get mixed signals. Even a minor rise in body heat can trigger sweating and a sense of intense warmth, usually in the face, neck, or chest. While hot flashes can vary from mild to severe, they often trace back to lower estrogen and its effects on the temperature-control center.

**Estrogen and the Brain**

Estrogen can affect the brain's chemical signals. Some brain areas have receptors that bind with estrogen, influencing moods, thinking, and even how nerves communicate. When estrogen levels drop, some women may notice changes in focus or memory. While this is not always severe, it can be noticeable enough for a woman to wonder if something is wrong. Research suggests that changes in estrogen can alter how the brain cells use energy, which may explain shifts in mental clarity or other mental tasks.

**Estrogen and Skin**

Skin often changes after menopause. Estrogen helps keep the skin more flexible by boosting collagen production. Collagen is a protein that keeps skin firm and elastic. As estrogen drops, collagen may decline too. This can lead to drier or thinner skin. Because of this, some women notice more wrinkles or fine lines. While this is normal aging, the drop in estrogen can speed up the process a bit.

---

# Progesterone's Role Outside of Pregnancy

Progesterone is often linked to pregnancy, as it prepares the uterus lining each month in case a fertilized egg attaches. But outside of its function in the uterus, progesterone has other roles too. It can influence mood, brain function, and even how the body handles fluid levels.

## Mood and Brain Effects

Progesterone can act on certain receptors in the brain that help regulate calm feelings. Some research suggests progesterone may support better rest. During the years leading up to menopause (perimenopause), progesterone may fluctuate more than estrogen. This can lead to uneven moods or trouble sleeping. By understanding progesterone's impact, a woman can see how these shifts might connect to anxiety or poor rest.

## Effects on Fluid Balance

Progesterone can act as a mild diuretic, helping the body excrete water and salt. When progesterone levels dip, some women may notice more fluid retention or bloating. This might explain why a woman's clothes feel tighter during certain phases of perimenopause.

---

# The Influence of Androgens

It might seem surprising, but women also produce male hormones, often called androgens. These include hormones like testosterone. While men produce more, women still have small amounts that can affect muscle strength, energy, and desire for intimacy.

## Testosterone in Women

A woman's ovaries and adrenal glands produce testosterone. Before menopause, testosterone contributes to muscle tone, mood, and sexual interest. As menopause nears, testosterone levels can also change, although not as sharply as estrogen. Still, the changes can be enough to make a woman notice differences in energy or a shift in sexual desire. Some women may also see an increase in facial hair, which can happen when the balance between estrogen and testosterone shifts.

## DHEA

Dehydroepiandrosterone (DHEA) is another androgen made by the adrenal glands. It can serve as a building block for making other hormones, including estrogen and testosterone. Some women have normal levels of DHEA throughout midlife, while others have lower levels. Studies on DHEA's effect are mixed, but changes in DHEA might add to shifts in mood and energy.

## Thyroid Hormones and Menopause

While thyroid hormones do not directly control menopause, they can affect how a woman feels. The thyroid gland helps manage metabolism, or how quickly the body uses energy. If thyroid hormone levels become too high or too low, it can lead to feelings of tiredness, weight changes, or mood swings. Because menopause already brings some of these signs, it is easy to confuse a thyroid problem with menopause. Checking thyroid function can be wise if a woman has unexplained weight changes, severe tiredness, or other unusual signs.

### Mixing Thyroid Problems with Menopause

If a woman thinks she is in menopause but her symptoms do not match the usual pattern—like extreme fatigue or very quick weight gain or loss—it might be a good idea to get a thyroid check. Sometimes, mild thyroid issues can become more noticeable around midlife. Proper treatment can make a big difference in how a woman feels.

## The Adrenal Glands' Role

The adrenal glands sit on top of the kidneys and produce several hormones, including cortisol (the "stress hormone") and small amounts of androgens. During menopause, the adrenal glands continue their usual tasks, but stress or chronic problems can lead to higher cortisol levels. This might increase tiredness or feelings of anxiety. While this is not directly menopause-related, the added stress of changes in midlife can put more strain on these glands.

### Stress, Cortisol, and Menopause

Cortisol can affect many aspects of daily life. If cortisol stays high, it can disrupt normal hormone balance even more. Women who experience a lot of stress during this phase may find their menopause signs feel more intense. Learning ways to manage stress can help keep cortisol levels in check and improve overall comfort.

## Hormones and the Immune System

Some research shows that estrogen interacts with the immune system. Estrogen can help regulate how the body reacts to infections or injuries. As estrogen levels drop after menopause, some women might notice changes in how often they get common illnesses, or how quickly they recover. More studies are needed, but there is a link between lower estrogen and certain shifts in immune activity. This does not mean that every woman will see a big difference, but it is worth knowing that hormones play a role here too.

## Impact on the Digestive System

Hormones can also influence how well the digestive tract works. For example, estrogen may help keep the lining of the gut healthy. Some women find that, during perimenopause or after menopause, they notice changes in bowel habits. These can include constipation or increased gas. Changing hormone levels may alter how quickly or slowly food moves through the intestines. If these changes are uncomfortable, it may be helpful to look at diet choices or check with a health expert.

## Summing Up Hormonal Effects

The human body is complex. Estrogen, progesterone, and other hormones interact in countless ways to keep processes in balance. During menopause, these interactions can shift quickly or slowly, which is why each woman's experience may differ. Here is a quick checklist of how each key hormone affects different parts of the body:

- **Estrogen:** Bones, skin, heart, brain, temperature control, and more.
- **Progesterone:** Mood stability, fluid balance, support for restful sleep.

- **Androgens (like testosterone)**: Muscle tone, sexual desire, energy.
- **Thyroid hormones**: Metabolism, energy use, weight changes (not strictly menopause-related, but can overlap).
- **Adrenal hormones (like cortisol)**: Stress management, energy, mood.

These hormones do not act alone. They often work together or counterbalance each other. When one hormone level falls, the body may try to adjust by raising or lowering others. This can lead to temporary periods of imbalance, which might be felt as hot flashes, mood swings, or fatigue.

## Monitoring Hormone Levels

Some women choose to have blood tests to measure their hormone levels around menopause. These tests can include:

- **FSH (Follicle-Stimulating Hormone)**: High levels usually signal menopause or perimenopause.
- **Estrogen levels (often called estradiol)**: Show how much the ovaries are producing.
- **Progesterone**: Hard to measure because it can vary day to day.
- **Thyroid panel**: Checks TSH (Thyroid-Stimulating Hormone), T3, and T4 levels to spot thyroid issues.
- **DHEA or testosterone**: Might be tested if there are signs of androgen imbalance.

While blood tests can offer clues, they are not the whole story. A woman's personal signs and how she feels often matter more than a single test result. Also, hormone levels can change rapidly, so a one-time test might not capture the entire picture. Some doctors prefer to base treatment on signs rather than repeated hormone tests.

## Managing Hormones Through Lifestyle Choices

Lifestyle changes can have a positive effect on hormone balance, even after menopause. It is not about restoring hormones to the levels of a 20-year-old, but rather about keeping the body in the best shape possible under new conditions.

1. **Stable Eating Habits**: Meals with a variety of nutrients (protein, healthy fats, vitamins, and minerals) can help the body maintain stable energy and reduce sudden blood sugar spikes.
2. **Regular Activity**: Activities like walking, swimming, or gentle strength exercises can help support muscle tone, bone health, and mood.
3. **Stress Management**: Activities like simple breathing exercises or listening to soothing music can help keep cortisol levels in check.
4. **Adequate Rest**: Getting enough sleep helps the body regulate hormone release and repair tissues.
5. **Avoiding Excessive Stimulants**: High caffeine intake or sugary snacks may worsen hot flashes or anxiety.
6. **Keeping Hydrated**: Drinking enough water can support many body functions, including digestion and temperature control.

---

## When Hormone Treatment May Help

If the normal changes in hormones cause severe signs that affect daily life, some women consider hormone treatments. These might include estrogen therapy or combined estrogen-progesterone therapy. However, these treatments have possible risks, so it is important to discuss them with a qualified health professional. We will talk more about hormone therapy in a later chapter, but know that such treatments aim to supplement the body's decreasing hormones and reduce troublesome signs.

---

## "Lesser-Known" Hormones Worth Mentioning

Aside from the well-known hormones, a few others may come up:

- **Relaxin**: This hormone helps loosen ligaments during pregnancy, and it can be present in smaller amounts at other times. Its levels are not a big factor in menopause, but changes in it could have mild effects on how flexible or stiff a woman's joints feel.
- **Melatonin**: Known for its role in sleep. It might shift with age, and lower levels can affect how easily a woman sleeps. Although it is not a direct menopause hormone, changes in sleep patterns are common during menopause, so melatonin could be relevant.

- **Leptin and Ghrelin**: These hormones help control appetite. While they are not strictly tied to menopause, changes in estrogen can affect body composition, and that can influence how leptin and ghrelin function. Some women notice increased hunger or different cravings during perimenopause.

# Myths About Hormones

1. **"All hormones stop during menopause."**
   Not true. The body still produces hormones, but the balance changes.
2. **"Once menopause hits, hormone levels never change again."**
   That is also not correct. Hormone levels can still shift in post-menopause, but usually at lower ranges than before.
3. **"Only estrogen matters in menopause."**
   While estrogen is major, other hormones like progesterone, testosterone, and adrenal hormones also play a part.

# Practical Steps for Hormone Awareness

- **Note Daily Changes**: Keep a simple log of mood, sleep quality, and energy. This can hint at hormonal changes.
- **Recognize Triggers**: Some women find that hot flashes are more frequent after a spicy meal or during stress.
- **Stay Informed**: Read about menopause from reliable sources, and ask health experts any questions.
- **Check Blood Tests if Needed**: If signs are confusing or severe, lab checks might help clarify.
- **Keep Communication Open**: Talking with loved ones about how you feel can reduce stress and help them understand.

# Conclusion

Hormones are key players in a woman's life before, during, and after menopause. While the changes in levels can bring challenges, knowing how these hormones interact with bones, skin, the immune system, and the brain can be empowering. It also helps to remember that hormones do not act alone—lifestyle choices, stress, and general health also influence how a woman experiences midlife changes.

This chapter took a closer look at each significant hormone and highlighted some that are not always discussed in typical menopause conversations. By seeing how these different chemical messengers support daily body functions, a woman can make better decisions about her diet, exercise routine, and when to ask a health professional for guidance.

In the next chapter, we will discuss the major body changes during menopause in more detail. We will look at how menopause can affect areas like the heart, digestive system, urinary tract, and more, beyond the basic signs people often talk about. This will provide a clearer picture of how broad the effects of menopause can be on overall health.

# Chapter 4: Major Body Changes During Menopause

Up to this point, we have looked at the stages of menopause and the roles of hormones in the body. Now, it is time to explore how menopause brings major changes to different systems. We will go beyond typical signs, like hot flashes and mood shifts, to examine the deeper changes happening in organs, tissues, and cells. Learning about these changes can guide a woman to take steps that may help her stay strong and healthy.

We will look at how menopause affects the heart and circulation, the digestive system, the urinary tract, the muscles, and the brain. Because estrogen levels drop, some shifts happen slowly over time, while others can show up quite suddenly. Each person's experience will be different, but understanding the possible effects can help a woman recognize what might be normal and what might need medical attention.

---

## Cardiovascular Changes

One of the more important changes after menopause involves the heart and blood vessels. Estrogen seems to have some protective effects on the walls of arteries. When estrogen levels fall, a woman may face a greater risk of heart and artery problems. This does not guarantee heart trouble, but the risk can increase compared to before menopause.

### Cholesterol and Arteries

Estrogen can influence the balance between good (HDL) cholesterol and bad (LDL) cholesterol. After menopause, LDL cholesterol may rise while HDL cholesterol can drop. If this goes unmanaged, plaques can build up in artery walls, raising the risk of heart attacks or strokes. Keeping an eye on cholesterol levels and working with a doctor can help keep the heart in good condition.

### Blood Pressure

Some women notice a rise in blood pressure after menopause. This might be partly linked to changes in hormones, but other factors—such as weight, salt intake, and stress—also matter. Tracking blood pressure numbers regularly, especially if there is a family history of high blood pressure, is a smart idea. If readings creep up, dietary changes or medications may help.

### Heart Rate and Rhythm

Lower estrogen levels might also affect the way nerves control the heart's rhythm. Some women may feel extra heartbeats or a pounding sensation (palpitations). Usually, these are harmless, but if they are happening a lot, it is best to see a health expert to rule out more serious problems.

## Effects on the Digestive System

Menopause can bring changes in how the digestive system processes food. As mentioned in the previous chapter, estrogen may help support a healthier gut lining. With lower estrogen, women might experience more bloating or constipation. Also, metabolism tends to slow down with age, which might lead to weight gain if a woman keeps eating the same amount of food as before.

### Changes in Gut Bacteria

Scientists are looking at the gut microbiome, which is the collection of bacteria and other microbes in the intestines. Research suggests that the drop in estrogen could shift the balance of these bacteria. While this is still being studied, an imbalance in gut bacteria can affect digestion, immune function, and even mood. Eating foods high in fiber and possibly adding probiotics or fermented foods might help keep the gut microbiome healthy.

### Heartburn and Acid Reflux

Some women find that heartburn or acid reflux becomes a bigger problem after menopause. This can be linked to weight changes or shifts in how the muscles around the food pipe work. If heartburn is frequent or severe, a health professional can suggest ways to manage it, such as adjusting mealtimes, using over-the-counter products, or prescribing medication.

## Urinary Tract Changes

The urinary tract includes the kidneys, the bladder, and the tube that carries urine out of the body (the urethra). Estrogen helps maintain the tissues in and around the urethra and bladder. After menopause, thinner tissues can lead to changes in bladder control or more frequent urges to use the bathroom.

### Bladder Control

A drop in estrogen may lower the strength of pelvic floor muscles. Some women notice they leak a small amount of urine when they sneeze or laugh. This is often called stress urinary incontinence. Pelvic floor exercises, which involve tightening and releasing the muscles around the bladder and vagina, can help a lot. If these exercises do not help, a doctor might have other suggestions.

### Urinary Tract Infections (UTIs)

Lower estrogen can also make the tissues of the urinary tract more prone to irritation or infection. Some women find they have more frequent UTIs after menopause. Drinking enough water and, in some cases, using a topical estrogen product (if recommended by a doctor) might reduce the risk of UTIs. Good personal hygiene is also key.

## Muscle and Joint Changes

Menopause can influence muscle mass and joint comfort. With lower estrogen, the body may not maintain muscle tissue as easily as before, and joints may feel stiffer or more achy.

### Loss of Muscle Mass

Age naturally brings a loss of muscle, but menopause can speed this up. Women may notice it is harder to keep strength or that they tire out more quickly when lifting items or climbing stairs. Combining protein-rich foods with strength-based exercises can help limit muscle loss. Even simple activities such as using light weights or doing exercises that use body weight can preserve muscle strength.

## Joint Pain and Stiffness

Some women report that their joints feel more uncomfortable or swollen after menopause. The exact reasons are not fully clear, but hormone changes can play a part in the health of the tissues around joints. Gentle stretches, heat therapy, and staying active can help reduce stiffness. If joint pain becomes intense, it may be worth checking with a health professional to see if there is an underlying condition like osteoarthritis.

---

# Brain and Cognitive Changes

We discussed in an earlier chapter that estrogen can affect the brain. After menopause, some women feel they are more forgetful or find it harder to focus. These changes are usually mild, but they can be frustrating.

## Memory and Focus

It is normal for memory to shift somewhat with age. Menopause can add to these changes, partly because of hormone shifts and partly because of issues like sleep trouble or stress. However, serious memory problems are not a typical part of menopause. If forgetfulness or confusion is severe, it is a good idea to rule out other causes, like thyroid disorders or certain nutrient deficiencies.

## Mood and Emotions

Menopause can also affect mood, sometimes bringing more irritability or worry. In addition, some women may notice changes in motivation or interest in daily tasks. These feelings can be managed through good sleep, healthy habits, or talking with a counselor if needed. Low levels of certain chemicals in the brain, combined with less estrogen, might explain these shifts.

---

# Skin, Hair, and Nail Changes

Many women talk about changes in their skin, hair, and nails during and after menopause. Estrogen keeps the skin more springy by boosting collagen and natural oils. When estrogen levels go down, these structures may change.

## Skin Changes

The skin might become thinner, drier, or itchier. Some women develop more lines, while others notice a change in texture. A gentle skin care routine that includes mild soaps, moisturizers, and sunscreen can help. Staying hydrated can also reduce dryness.

## Hair Thinning or Loss

Hair can thin out on the scalp or become more fragile. A rise in the relative effect of male hormones can lead to hair thinning patterns some women do not like. Meanwhile, some may notice more hair growth on the chin or upper lip. Using products designed for thinning hair and talking with a health professional can help manage these changes.

## Nail Brittleness

Nails might break more easily or develop ridges. This can be linked to lower levels of hormones as well as changes in nutrient absorption. Eating foods rich in vitamins and minerals, like leafy greens or nuts, might help maintain healthier nails.

---

# Changes in Body Composition

Another major shift involves where the body stores fat. After menopause, many women find that fat collects around the waist rather than on the hips and thighs. This can be related to changes in insulin sensitivity, cortisol levels, and the reduced levels of estrogen.

### Waistline Increases

A thicker waist can raise health risks linked to heart issues or blood sugar problems. Some women notice this happens even if they have not changed their eating habits. Regular physical movement and a balanced diet can help manage these changes. It is not always about becoming very thin, but rather maintaining a healthy range for one's body type.

### Muscle-to-Fat Ratio

Because the body may be losing muscle, the portion of fat could rise. This can change how a woman's shape looks and lead to weight gain. Even small changes in activity, like taking the stairs instead of the elevator, can add up over time. Strengthening exercises, even if done a few times a week, can help maintain muscle mass.

---

## Vision and Eye Health

Estrogen affects many tissues, and the eyes are no exception. Some women notice drier eyes or changes in vision around midlife. Eye dryness may come from reduced tear production. Using over-the-counter lubricating eye drops can be helpful if dryness causes discomfort.

### Eye Pressure and Age

As women age, the pressure inside the eye might go up. While this may not be directly caused by menopause, it is still good to have regular eye exams. Early detection of issues like glaucoma can save eyesight.

---

## Dental and Gum Health

Hormone levels can affect the health of the gums. Some women experience a higher chance of gum bleeding or inflammation after menopause. Good dental care—regular brushing, flossing, and dental check-ups—can help protect the mouth. In some cases, dryness in the mouth can occur, which can also affect oral health. Drinking enough water and using special mouthwashes or rinses may reduce dryness.

## Fatigue and Energy Levels

Menopause can sometimes bring a sense of weariness. This might be due to poor sleep from night sweats, or it can be because of fluctuating hormones. In addition, changes in mood and emotional stress can leave a woman feeling drained.

### Sleep Interruptions

Many women mention that hot flashes or night sweats wake them up multiple times a night. This broken sleep can result in tiredness during the day. Keeping the bedroom cool, wearing loose-fitting sleepwear, and avoiding heavy blankets can help. If sleep loss becomes severe, speaking with a doctor about possible treatments may make a real difference.

### Checking for Other Causes

Fatigue can also come from anemia, thyroid issues, or problems like sleep apnea. If a woman feels constantly exhausted even with good sleep habits, it is wise to get tested to rule out other conditions. Correcting an underlying problem can improve well-being in a big way.

## Emotional and Social Factors

Major body changes can also bring emotional challenges. Some women feel less confident when they see changes in their hair or waistline. Others feel pressure from family or work responsibilities while also managing menopause. This can all build up and lead to stress.

### Body Image Concerns

New wrinkles or weight changes can make some women feel upset about aging. It may help to remember that changes over time are normal. If a woman feels overwhelmed by these concerns, talking with a trusted friend or counselor can offer support. Finding comfortable clothing and choosing grooming routines that help a woman feel at ease can also help her cope with outward changes.

### Managing Social Expectations

Sometimes, people around a woman going through menopause might not fully understand these changes. They might expect her to maintain the same energy level or emotional reactions she had before. Discussing menopause with friends or family in a calm way can help them learn what is happening. This reduces misunderstandings and can lead to more empathy.

## Preventive Measures and Check-Ups

Because menopause can raise the risk of certain health problems, it is vital to have regular check-ups and screenings. These might include:

- **Bone density scans**: To look for early signs of osteoporosis.
- **Heart health checks**: Including blood pressure and cholesterol tests.
- **Routine blood work**: To spot any nutrient deficits or thyroid issues.
- **Eye exams**: Especially if changes in vision occur.

Early detection can make a big difference in handling any concerns that appear after menopause. Some doctors also recommend certain vaccines to help guard against infections that might be more troublesome in older age.

## Home and Daily Life Adjustments

Women can take various steps at home to cope with changes in their bodies:

1. **Set a Regular Sleep Schedule**: Going to bed and waking up at the same times each day helps.
2. **Adjust Your Wardrobe**: Lighter layers allow you to remove clothing if you get too warm.
3. **Optimize Your Diet**: Foods rich in calcium, vitamin D, and other nutrients help.

4. **Try Gentle Exercises**: This can keep joints flexible and muscles strong.
5. **Stay Hydrated**: Drinking enough water can aid digestion and reduce dryness in eyes, skin, and mouth.
6. **Consider Support Groups**: Talking with others going through the same changes can reduce stress.

---

# Looking Forward

Even though menopause can bring a wide range of body changes, many women go on to have fulfilling lives and maintain good health. Some signs or concerns can decrease over time as the body settles into its new hormone levels. Others may need regular attention, like checking bone strength or heart health. The most important thing is awareness—knowing what is happening so a woman can respond in ways that feel right for her.

In the next chapter, we will look at physical shifts like hot flashes, muscle aches, and sleep disturbances, as well as how to manage them. There, we will focus on straightforward strategies that can be done at home or with the help of professionals. That discussion will build on the knowledge from this chapter, connecting the body changes we have learned about to everyday activities and health habits.

---

# Chapter 4 Summary

In this chapter, we explored the major body changes that can happen during menopause, including impacts on the heart, digestive system, urinary tract, muscles, brain, skin, and more. We learned how lower estrogen might raise the risk of heart problems and how it can affect digestion, bladder control, and bone health. We also covered changes in body composition, eye health, and oral care. By recognizing these changes, women can better handle problems such as weight shifts, hot flashes, and fatigue.

Understanding these physical changes is part of taking action to stay healthy. This might mean adjusting diet, adding consistent exercise, or seeking advice from doctors. Although menopause can bring significant shifts, knowledge and good daily habits can reduce difficulties and help a woman adapt.

# Chapter 5: Physical Shifts and How to Manage Them

In the earlier chapters, we discussed hormones and the different changes that happen in a woman's body as she approaches and passes through menopause. Now, let us focus on specific physical signs and how to manage them in daily life. Menopause can bring a wide range of shifts that affect sleep, comfort, and overall well-being. Each woman is different, so not everyone will have the same signs. Still, it helps to be prepared and to know about simple and practical ways to handle these changes.

This chapter will look at hot flashes, muscle and joint aches, changes in body temperature, headaches, and how to stay comfortable. We will also discuss some less common physical signs, such as increased skin sensitivity or a change in how the senses of taste or smell work. By knowing ways to manage these signs, a woman can keep a sense of stability in her everyday routine.

## Hot Flashes and Night Sweats

Hot flashes and night sweats are among the most well-known signs of menopause. Many women find them uncomfortable or even embarrassing, especially if they happen in public. Luckily, there are ways to reduce how strong and how frequent they are.

### Why Do They Happen?

Hot flashes and night sweats stem from changes in how the body controls temperature. With lower levels of estrogen, the temperature-regulating center in the brain becomes more sensitive. Small increases in body heat can lead to the sensation of extreme warmth. In night sweats, this occurs during sleep, leading a woman to wake up sweaty and possibly chilled afterward.

### Strategies for Reducing Hot Flashes

1. **Cool Environment**: Keep rooms at a cooler temperature. Using a fan or opening a window can help.
2. **Breathable Clothing**: Choose fabrics like cotton and loose-fitting styles that allow heat to escape.

3. **Layering**: Wear clothing in layers so you can remove something if you feel too warm.
4. **Avoid Triggers**: Some find that hot or spicy foods, alcohol, and caffeine make hot flashes worse. Identify your triggers and limit them if possible.
5. **Relaxation Methods**: Breathing exercises, light stretching, or listening to calm music can help slow the heart rate and reduce the intensity of a hot flash.

## Handling Night Sweats

- **Cool Bedding**: Use cotton sheets and light blankets. A mattress pad made from cooling materials may also help.
- **Light Sleepwear**: A simple cotton nightgown or pajamas are easier on the skin than heavy or synthetic fabrics.
- **Hydration**: Keep water next to the bed to sip if you wake up overheated.
- **Pre-Bed Routine**: Avoid very hot showers just before bed, and steer clear of late-night spicy dinners. A cooler meal closer to bedtime may reduce night sweats.

---

# Muscle and Joint Aches

Some women experience more stiffness or achiness in their muscles and joints around menopause. This can make it harder to do daily tasks, such as climbing stairs or carrying groceries. Below are some suggestions for staying comfortable and mobile.

## Gentle Movement and Stretching

Regular movement can help keep joints loose and muscles strong. Consider low-impact activities like walking or simple at-home stretching. Even taking a short walk around the block each day can reduce stiffness. Using light hand weights for a few sets of basic exercises can help maintain muscle mass.

## Temperature-Based Comfort

Applying warm packs to stiff joints may help loosen them before exercise. Some women find relief from applying a cool pack after activity if the joints feel inflamed or sore. Experiment to see which temperature helps you most.

## Posture Checks

Poor posture can worsen aches. If you spend a lot of time sitting, make sure your chair provides support for your lower back. Keep both feet on the floor and avoid slouching. If you work on a computer, adjust the screen so it is at eye level. This reduces strain on the neck and shoulders.

## When to Seek Help

If joint pain or muscle aches become intense or do not improve with simple measures, talk to a health professional. They can check if there is an underlying cause like arthritis. Physical therapy might also help. Strengthening certain muscle groups can support the joints and minimize pain.

---

# Changes in Body Temperature Beyond Hot Flashes

Though hot flashes are common, some women also notice they feel colder than usual at times. Shifts in hormone levels can make the body's temperature regulation unpredictable. You might feel warm one minute and chilly the next.

## Layering and Adjusting Clothing

Carrying a light sweater or shawl is helpful. You can put it on if you suddenly feel chilled. Layering is handy for handling sudden warmth or cold. This tactic is especially useful in workplaces or public buildings where you cannot control the thermostat.

## Staying Well-Hydrated

Drinking enough water helps maintain healthy blood flow, which can stabilize body temperature. Mild dehydration might make you feel colder or hotter than normal. Aiming for around 6-8 glasses of water a day is a good start, but needs may vary based on factors like exercise and climate.

---

# Headaches and Migraines

Some women notice an increase in headaches or migraines as hormone levels change. Hormone fluctuations can trigger blood vessels in the brain to tighten or widen, leading to different types of headaches.

## Identifying Triggers

Jot down notes on when headaches occur and what might have triggered them—certain foods, stress, bright lights, or strong smells. Recognizing your triggers can help you avoid them in the future.

## Relaxation and Over-the-Counter Options

If you have mild headaches, lying down in a dark, quiet room can help. Over-the-counter pain relievers might offer short-term relief. However, if headaches grow worse or happen frequently, a health expert can suggest advanced strategies, possibly including prescription medicines or preventive treatments.

---

# Skin Sensitivity and Changes in Senses

Menopause can sometimes bring heightened skin sensitivity. Fabrics that never bothered you before might now feel itchy or rough. In rare cases, some women also notice changes in how they taste or smell things.

## Skin Sensitivity

- **Gentle Cleansers**: Use mild soaps free of harsh chemicals. A fragrance-free moisturizer can help prevent dryness and itching.
- **Patch Test Products**: If you decide to try a new lotion or soap, test it on a small area first to see if your skin reacts.
- **Soft Fabrics**: Choose cotton, bamboo, or other natural fabrics that breathe well. Avoid tight clothing that can rub and irritate the skin.

### Changes in Taste or Smell

Some women find their sense of taste becomes less sharp, or that some foods now have a different flavor. Others might notice sensitivity to strong smells like perfumes or cleaning products. If these changes affect your daily life, consider using fragrance-free products and cooking with milder spices. If your sense of taste or smell drops suddenly, it might be a good idea to talk with a health professional to rule out other causes.

---

## Maintaining Comfort During Daily Activities

When physical signs of menopause surface, they can affect everyday life, from driving to shopping to cooking at home. Below are suggestions for staying comfortable during day-to-day tasks.

### Driving

If hot flashes strike while you are driving, it can be distracting. Keeping a small fan that plugs into the car's power outlet or opening windows can bring quick relief. Dress in breathable layers so that you can cool down easily if needed.

### Working

Desk jobs can be uncomfortable if you are dealing with hot flashes or muscle aches. Consider a small desk fan if your workplace allows it. Get up and stretch every hour or so to reduce stiffness. If possible, talk with your supervisor or human resources about any needed adjustments, like a more comfortable chair or a flexible schedule for short breaks.

### Shopping and Errands

Plan shopping trips during cooler parts of the day if you tend to get overheated. Bring a water bottle. Wear shoes that support your feet well, since muscle and joint aches can feel worse if you spend a long time on your feet. If needed, take short breaks and sit on a bench or in your car before continuing.

# Supporting Nutrition for Physical Comfort

A balanced diet can help reduce certain physical signs or at least keep them from getting worse. Here are some focused ideas:

1. **Protein-Rich Foods**: Helps maintain muscle mass. Good examples include lean poultry, fish, beans, eggs, and nuts.
2. **Calcium and Vitamin D**: Protects bones and may reduce aches. Dairy products, fortified cereals, and leafy greens can help, alongside moderate sun exposure for vitamin D.
3. **Omega-3 Fatty Acids**: These can support joint health and possibly lower inflammation. Found in fish (such as salmon), walnuts, and flaxseeds.
4. **Magnesium**: Can aid muscle relaxation and reduce certain types of headaches. Good sources include almonds, spinach, and avocados.
5. **Limit Caffeine and Alcohol**: Both can worsen hot flashes and disrupt sleep.

---

# Physical Techniques for Relief

In addition to daily habits, there are hands-on methods that may offer relief from menopause-related discomforts.

## Massage

Gentle massage can help ease tense muscles and improve circulation. Some women find that massaging the shoulders or lower back helps with aches. If you can, try working with a trained massage therapist who is aware of menopause issues. Self-massage at home is also an option, using a tennis ball against a wall to roll away tension points.

## Simple Breathing Exercises

When you feel a hot flash beginning, or if you have a headache, deep, slow breaths can steady the heart rate and help calm the mind. A simple way is to inhale slowly through the nose, count to four, then exhale through the mouth over a count of four. Repeat several times.

### Gentle Stretch Sessions

A short stretch session in the morning and before bedtime can help reduce stiffness. Focus on major muscle groups: arms, legs, back, and neck. Movements should be slow and steady. Avoid bouncing. This can be part of a longer routine or just a quick five-minute practice to loosen up.

### Warm or Cool Baths

A warm bath can relax tense muscles. If you feel overheated from hot flashes, a lukewarm or slightly cool bath or shower might help bring down your core temperature. Add gentle bath products if desired, but steer clear of anything with harsh chemicals that might irritate the skin.

---

# The Role of Rest and Sleep

Poor or interrupted sleep can make physical menopause signs feel worse. For example, if you are tired, you may be more likely to feel aches. Hot flashes might also seem more intense when you lack enough rest. Making sure you get a good night's sleep is crucial for overall health and resilience.

### Improving Sleep Quality

- **Regular Schedule**: Go to bed and wake up at the same time each day, including weekends.
- **Cool Bedroom**: Use a fan or air conditioner to create a cooler environment.
- **Calming Activities**: Avoid heavy meals, bright screens, or stressful discussions right before bedtime.
- **Limit Late-Night Caffeine**: Even if you had caffeine earlier in the day, it might keep you awake later than you realize.

If sleep troubles become severe, it might help to consult a health expert who can guide you on possible sleep aids, therapies, or other interventions.

---

# Tracking Your Physical Changes

Keeping track of when signs occur and what might make them better or worse can guide you and your health professional. This does not have to be fancy—just a small notebook or a note-taking app on your phone.

## What to Record

- **Dates and Times**: Note when hot flashes, headaches, or aches happen.
- **Possible Triggers**: Did you eat something spicy? Were you stressed out?
- **Intensity**: Mild, moderate, or severe?
- **Relief Methods**: What helped? A cool drink, rest, or a pain reliever?

Patterns might emerge over time, helping you avoid triggers or choose the best coping methods.

---

# Addressing Less Common Physical Shifts

Menopause can also bring some surprises:

1. **Changes in Nails**: Some women see brittle or ridged nails. Keep them trimmed and use a gentle nail oil if dryness is a problem.
2. **Tingling Sensations**: Occasional tingling in the hands or feet, sometimes called paresthesia, might happen. If it is frequent or intense, check with a health professional to rule out nerve issues.
3. **Balance Issues**: Hormonal changes and aging can affect balance. Simple exercises that focus on stable footing, such as standing on one foot next to a chair for support, can help improve balance over time.

---

# Benefits of Shared Support

Sometimes, the best help for physical menopause signs is learning from others who have faced them. Consider joining a support group, either in person or online. Hearing about tactics that helped other women handle hot flashes at work or manage daily errands can give you new ideas. Support groups can also be reassuring if you feel overwhelmed or confused about physical shifts that do not get talked about much in everyday conversation.

## Handling Personal Care and Hygiene

Physical changes during menopause may call for slight alterations in personal care. For example, you might notice more dryness or discomfort in certain areas. Using gentle, pH-balanced products can reduce irritation. Some women also find that they need to change their undergarments' material to something that allows the skin to breathe better.

### Grooming Routines

Because of hair thinning or changes in skin texture, grooming might take a bit of extra planning. Some women switch to milder shampoos or add scalp treatments that encourage healthy hair. For skin care, focusing on sun protection, gentle exfoliation, and a good moisturizer can maintain smoother skin. These routines do not have to be expensive or complicated—small daily habits can have a big impact.

## Balancing Activity and Rest

When dealing with menopause signs, it is key to find the right level of daily activity. Too little movement might make stiffness and aches worse. Too much intense exercise can lead to soreness or overheating. Balance is the key. Some women benefit from short, repeated bouts of activity rather than a single long session. For instance:

- **Morning**: A quick walk around the neighborhood.
- **Lunch Break**: Simple stretches in the office or a brisk 10-minute walk.
- **Evening**: Light yoga-like routine or a gentle activity before dinner.

Listening to your body's signals helps you avoid overdoing it.

# When Professional Care Is Needed

While many menopause signs can be managed at home, there are times when seeking professional help is wise:

1. **Severe Hot Flashes**: If they happen many times a day and affect your quality of life, your doctor may suggest hormone therapy or other treatments.
2. **Intense Muscle/Joint Pain**: This might not be just menopause. There could be an underlying condition like arthritis or an autoimmune issue.
3. **Long-Term Headaches**: Recurring migraines or severe headaches might require a neurologist's evaluation.
4. **Consistent Unusual Changes**: Any persistent or unexplained physical change should be checked out to rule out more serious problems.

---

# Practical Tools and Gadgets

Some women find relief through tools designed to ease physical changes:

- **Cooling Towels**: Specially designed towels stay cool for a while after being soaked in water, handy for hot flashes or hot weather.
- **Handheld Fans**: Battery-operated or manual fans can bring quick relief in public spaces.
- **Moisture-Wicking Clothing**: Athletic or specialized sleepwear can draw sweat away from the body more effectively.
- **Supportive Shoes**: Helps reduce foot and joint pain if you walk or stand a lot.

---

# Positive Self-Care Mindset

Menopause does bring changes, but a person can still stay active and comfortable. Instead of thinking of these signs as permanent barriers, view them as signals that the body's needs are shifting. By paying attention and responding with small adjustments—like wearing cooler clothing, adding a short walk to your day, or modifying your diet—you can continue enjoying daily life.

It also helps to stay connected with friends, relatives, or mentors who have gone through menopause. They may offer practical tips that worked for them. Above all, remember that you are not alone, and there is no single "right" or "wrong" way to handle these physical signs. Your focus should be on finding what brings you relief and supports your well-being.

## Chapter 5 Summary

Menopause can lead to hot flashes, night sweats, muscle aches, joint stiffness, and various other physical shifts. Each woman experiences these in her own way, but there are many practical tips to handle them. Simple actions like layering clothes, checking posture, staying hydrated, and tracking triggers can go a long way in providing relief. Remember that proper rest and balanced nutrition are also vital during this time.

Beyond everyday measures, there are tools and professional approaches if signs become severe. Whether it is a cooling towel, a desk fan at work, a mild pain reliever for headaches, or physical therapy for ongoing joint issues, the goal is to maintain comfort. Staying aware of your body's changes and seeking help when needed are the keys to handling menopause's physical shifts. In the next chapter, we will explore how menopause can affect emotions, including mood swings and changes in mental well-being, and what methods can help keep things in balance.

# Chapter 6: Emotional Changes and Balance

Menopause does not only bring physical changes. It also plays a big role in how a woman feels emotionally. Shifts in hormone levels can lead to mood swings, feelings of sadness or worry, and changes in self-esteem. This chapter will look at why emotional shifts happen during menopause, how to cope, and where to find support. We will also discuss relationships—both at home and work—and ways to keep them healthy in the face of emotional ups and downs.

While emotional changes can be confusing or even frightening, it is important to remember that they are often a normal response to changing hormone levels and life circumstances. With the right awareness and tools, a woman can handle these feelings and remain connected to those who care about her. Learning ways to find balance can make a huge difference in daily well-being.

---

## Why Emotional Shifts Occur

Emotional changes during menopause can be traced to a mix of factors:

1. **Hormones**: As estrogen and progesterone levels go down, chemical signals in the brain shift. These fluctuations can affect mood-regulating substances like serotonin.
2. **Physical Discomfort**: Hot flashes, sleep troubles, and aches can make a woman feel stressed or cranky.
3. **Life Events**: Midlife often coincides with aging parents, children leaving home, or changes in a career. These events can add stress.
4. **Self-Perception**: Menopause can cause some women to feel uncertain about aging and their identity.

All these factors weave together, shaping a woman's emotional experience. While these feelings can be strong, many strategies and resources can help lessen their impact.

# Common Emotional Signs

Each woman's emotional pattern is unique, but some common themes emerge:

1. **Mood Swings**: Feeling content one moment, then sad or annoyed the next.
2. **Sadness or Low Mood**: This can range from feeling mildly down to symptoms that resemble depression.
3. **Anxiety and Worry**: Some may feel a constant sense of unease or fear about the future.
4. **Irritability**: Trivial things may cause frustration more quickly than before.
5. **Loss of Motivation**: A lack of interest in daily tasks or hobbies previously enjoyed.

These changes can feel unsettling, especially if you are not aware they may be linked to menopause. Recognizing the connection can help you be kinder to yourself and seek better coping methods.

---

# Strategies for Emotional Balance

Below are ways to foster emotional balance. Each person will find different combinations that work best, so it helps to experiment and remain open to new ideas.

## 1. A Support Network

Reaching out to people who are understanding is often the first step in handling emotional changes:

- **Friends and Family**: Explain that you might need more patience or a listening ear.
- **Support Groups**: Local or online groups where women share experiences about menopause. Hearing similar stories can reduce the sense of isolation.
- **Professional Help**: Counselors, therapists, or social workers can offer tools for handling worry or sadness. They also provide a confidential space to talk about personal fears.

## 2. Mindful Techniques

Though there are many approaches, simple practices can calm the mind:

- **Slow Breathing**: If you feel panic or heavy worry, pause and take several slow breaths in and out.
- **Short Breaks**: Give yourself permission to rest when anxiety or irritability spikes. Even a five-minute break can refresh your mood.
- **Focus on the Present**: Try to bring your attention to what you are doing right now—whether it is washing dishes or walking the dog—rather than worrying about past or future events.

## 3. Maintain a Routine

A steady daily routine can bring order to feelings that seem out of control:

- **Regular Sleep Schedule**: Going to bed and waking up at consistent times supports mood balance.
- **Meal Times**: Eating at similar times each day stabilizes blood sugar, which can help with emotional steadiness.
- **Physical Activity**: A short walk or simple stretching can lift mood and reduce stress.

---

# Handling Anger and Irritability

Some women find themselves snapping at loved ones more often. This can lead to guilt or shame, which may worsen mood swings. Here are suggestions for handling irritability:

1. **Identify Triggers**: Think about what sets you off. Is it certain noises, clutter in the home, or feeling rushed at work?
2. **Plan Ahead**: If you know certain situations test your patience, try to reduce them. For example, you might shop at quieter hours or keep the home less cluttered.
3. **Release Tension**: Find healthy ways to release frustration, such as writing in a journal or doing a few quick exercises.
4. **Apologize When Needed**: If you lose your temper with someone, a simple sorry can mend relationships and relieve guilt.

# Dealing with Sadness or Low Mood

Feeling sad or down can be a normal part of menopause for some women. Changes in hormones, body image worries, and life stress can combine to weigh a person down.

1. **Identify Mental Health Needs**: If sadness is constant or severe, a counselor or doctor can assess whether it is linked to depression. This is important because depression is treatable, and professional support can help.
2. **Build a Hope List**: Make a short list of activities or goals you look forward to—a hobby, a trip to a local park, or a project at home. Looking ahead to positive events helps balance sadness.
3. **Light Therapy**: If low mood is strong during winter months, bright light therapy might help. Speak with a health expert to see if this is right for you.
4. **Focus on Achievements**: Each day, write down one or two small achievements. It could be cooking a nice meal, cleaning part of the house, or calling a friend. This shifts the mind toward positive actions.

---

# Anxiety and Worry

Menopause can increase worry, whether about health, aging, or family. Prolonged worry may lead to sleepless nights and tension in the neck or shoulders.

### Short-Term Methods

- **Grounding Technique**: Name five things you can see, four you can feel, three you can hear, two you can smell, and one you can taste. This brings you into the present moment.
- **Write It Down**: Journaling fears can lessen their intensity.

### Longer-Term Approaches

- **Counseling**: A professional can guide you in shaping healthier thought patterns.

- **Relaxation Training**: This might involve gentle muscle relaxation or guided audio tracks that promote calm.
- **Setting Limits**: If watching the news triggers anxiety, limit how much you watch. If certain social media feeds worsen your worry, adjust your usage.

---

# Changing Family and Social Roles

Midlife often brings changes in household dynamics. Children may become teenagers or leave home. Parents might need extra care. These shifts can trigger mixed emotions—relief, sadness, worry, or guilt.

1. **Family Talks**: Talk with family members about how you feel. If you are caring for aging parents, share tasks with siblings or other relatives.
2. **Clear Boundaries**: If adult children return home, set guidelines about finances, chores, or daily routines.
3. **Plan for the Future**: Talk about retirement options or where you want to live. Making plans can reduce worry about uncertainty.

---

# Self-Image and Confidence

Menopause may alter how some women see themselves. Changing body shape, wrinkles, or hair thinning can affect confidence. However, many women also discover new forms of self-assurance with the knowledge and experience they have gained over time.

## Building Confidence

- **New Interests**: Exploring a hobby or skill can create a sense of purpose and achievement.
- **Wardrobe Adjustments**: Wear clothes that fit comfortably and make you feel good. Sometimes, picking styles that suit your current shape can refresh your outlook.
- **Positive Self-Talk**: Be kind to yourself. Avoid negative labels. Remind yourself of your strengths, whether they are career skills, creative talents, or strong friendships.

# Healthy Communication in Relationships

Emotional shifts can strain relationships if they are not understood or discussed. Partners, children, and friends might not realize what you are going through.

## Talk Openly

Explain menopause to those close to you. Let them know that mood swings can happen, and that it is not their fault. If you feel comfortable, give examples: "I might get upset more quickly these days, but it's something I'm working on. Thank you for being patient."

## Request Support

If you need space or help with tasks, say so. If night sweats keep you up, you might ask your partner to adjust bedding or open a window before bed. Sometimes, simply having a loved one listen can reduce feelings of isolation or frustration.

---

# Work-Life Concerns

Menopause often arrives at a time when a woman might be in the middle of a career or considering a change. Emotional shifts can make work more challenging, especially if hot flashes or mood swings occur on the job.

## Handling Stress at Work

- **Work Breaks**: Take short breaks to regroup if anxiety or irritability rises. A brief walk or some deep breaths can reset your mood.
- **Support at Work**: If you trust a colleague or supervisor, discuss any needed accommodations. This might be as simple as having a fan or flexible break times.
- **Set Clear Limits**: Avoid taking on every project or working extra hours if stress is high. Saying no to extra tasks can protect your emotional health.
- **Plan Transitions**: If you are thinking about part-time work or shifting roles, gather information and talk to a career counselor. Planning can reduce worries about an uncertain future.

# Lifestyle Habits That Support Emotional Well-Being

Your daily habits can either feed negative emotions or help calm them.

1. **Regular Physical Activity**: Exercise releases feel-good chemicals in the brain. Even 20 minutes a day of gentle movement can boost mood.
2. **Nutritious Meals**: Large swings in blood sugar can affect energy and mood. Balanced meals with proteins, healthy fats, and complex carbs can keep you on a more even keel.
3. **Limit Stimulants**: High amounts of caffeine can raise anxiety, and too much alcohol can disrupt sleep and worsen low mood.
4. **Relaxing Pastimes**: Activities like listening to music, reading, or light crafting can ease stress and distract from negative thoughts.

---

# Recognizing Serious Concerns

While some emotional shifts are normal, it is important to spot signs that more help is needed:

- **Persistent Sadness**: Lasting more than two weeks and not improving.
- **Severe Anxiety**: Ongoing worry that disrupts daily life or leads to panic attacks.
- **Thoughts of Harming Yourself or Others**: This is a crisis sign. Seek immediate help from a health professional or a hotline.
- **Problems Functioning**: If mood issues keep you from working, caring for yourself, or handling normal tasks, it is time to seek professional support.

A doctor or mental health expert can determine if you are facing a clinical problem such as major depression or an anxiety disorder. Treatments could include talk therapy, medicine, or a combination.

---

# Simple Exercises to Ease Emotional Pressure

## Quick Gratitude Check

Take one minute each day to name something you are thankful for. It could be a comfortable bed, a pet, or a kind friend. This practice can shift focus from the negative to the positive.

## Body Scan

Sit or lie down in a quiet space. Slowly bring your attention to each part of the body, starting with the toes and moving up to the head. Notice any tension and gently release it. This can bring calm and a sense of awareness.

## Progressive Muscle Tensing

Clench one muscle group for a few seconds, then release. Move through your arms, legs, and torso. This can help you recognize when you are holding tension without realizing it.

# The Role of Professional Guidance

Therapists and counselors who specialize in midlife issues can offer valuable advice. They may use methods like cognitive behavioral techniques, which help reframe negative thoughts, or interpersonal therapy, which focuses on relationship patterns. Some health professionals might also suggest medicines or supplements if the emotional shifts are severe.

It is wise to keep an open mind about professional care. Many women find that short-term therapy sessions give them new skills to manage mood swings, worry, or sadness. Others prefer long-term counseling, especially if there are ongoing stress factors in their lives.

# Building Resilience Over Time

Menopause can be a period of self-discovery as well as emotional stress. Building resilience means growing stronger and more adaptable to life's changes:

1. **Learn from Setbacks**: If a strategy fails (for example, you try a relaxation method and it does not help), think of it as data. It is just showing you a different path might work better.
2. **Stay Connected**: Isolation can increase negative thoughts. Talk to friends, join social groups, or volunteer for local causes. Connection fosters a sense of purpose.

3. **Recognize Personal Growth**: Overcoming tough emotional days can make you feel proud of yourself. Notice small improvements in how you handle stress.
4. **Health Checkups**: Keeping up with regular medical and mental health checkups is a part of building resilience. Catching issues early can save bigger problems later.

## Combining Physical and Emotional Care

Emotional well-being is closely tied to physical health. If you are dealing with hot flashes, muscle aches, or sleep trouble, these can increase emotional sensitivity. Addressing physical symptoms often leads to better emotional stability. Likewise, improving emotional habits can lessen the intensity of physical signs. For instance, if you reduce chronic worry, you might find that your headaches or sleep disruptions improve.

## Chapter 6 Summary

Emotional changes during menopause can include mood swings, sadness, worry, and low confidence. These shifts can stem from a blend of hormone changes, life events, and self-image. While they can be challenging, many coping methods exist—ranging from support networks and mindful techniques to therapy and healthy lifestyle choices. Recognizing triggers, sticking to a stable routine, and opening up to friends, family, or professionals can help maintain balance.

Remember that not all emotional changes are resolved quickly or easily. Patience and steady effort can lead to greater self-understanding and inner strength. In the next chapters, we will explore more topics related to menopause, such as sleep concerns, weight changes, and bone health. Each part of this book aims to give you more insights and tools for handling the varied aspects of menopause, so you can find solutions that fit your life.

# Chapter 7: Sleep Concerns and Energy Levels

When a woman enters menopause, changes in sleep can be very common. Some women experience more interrupted rest at night, find it harder to fall asleep, or wake up much earlier than usual. Others feel so tired during the day that simple tasks become draining. All of this can stem from the shift in hormone levels, along with stress, hot flashes, and other factors that affect comfort. This chapter takes a detailed look at what can happen to sleep and energy levels during menopause, as well as practical ways to improve both.

## Understanding Why Sleep Changes

### Hormones Affect the Sleep Cycle

Before menopause, steady levels of hormones—especially estrogen and progesterone—help support stable sleep rhythms. As these hormones shift, the body's internal clock can become a bit unsettled. Some women find themselves suddenly wide awake at 3 a.m., while others have problems getting to sleep in the first place. Here are key points about how hormones can shape sleep:

1. **Estrogen and Body Temperature**: Estrogen helps regulate body temperature to some degree. With lower estrogen, you may sweat more at night or experience sudden warmth, often called night sweats. Waking up hot or sweaty can prevent deep sleep.
2. **Progesterone's Calming Influence**: Progesterone can support relaxation for some women. When it goes down, the brain may not enter a relaxed state as easily, raising the chances of tossing and turning at bedtime.
3. **Stress Hormones**: Menopause can also be a stressful time, which can cause higher levels of cortisol (the stress hormone). Elevated cortisol makes it tougher to wind down.

### Physical Discomfort

Physical issues like joint aches, muscle tightness, or a full bladder (if you are dealing with urinary changes) can interrupt sleep. If you are already waking with night sweats, the added discomfort from these other factors can lead to frequent awakenings. These broken sleep patterns can lower the total amount of restful sleep each night.

## Emotional Factors

During menopause, the mind may be busy with worries about health, family, or personal goals. Anxiety can make it hard to relax. If you spend time in bed thinking over problems, you might start associating bedtime with tension. This loop can make falling asleep or staying asleep more difficult.

---

# Common Sleep Problems During Menopause

1. **Trouble Falling Asleep**: It might feel like the mind is racing, or the body is too restless to settle down.
2. **Frequent Awakenings**: You may drift off but then wake up several times each night.
3. **Early Morning Waking**: Some women find they wake at 4 or 5 a.m. and cannot go back to sleep, even though they are still tired.
4. **Unrefreshed Sleep**: You might sleep for several hours but wake feeling as though you barely rested.
5. **Snoring or Sleep Apnea**: In some cases, weight changes or muscle tone changes in the throat can lead to snoring or even sleep apnea, a condition where breathing stops briefly during sleep.

---

# Impact on Daytime Energy

## Mood and Concentration

A lack of solid rest can affect mood, concentration, and quick thinking. Tasks that were once easy may feel harder because your brain is running on low energy. Irritability or sadness might also increase when you do not get enough sleep, feeding into a cycle of tension.

## Physical Fatigue

Aches and low stamina can become worse when you are sleep-deprived. Even minor tasks like washing dishes, walking upstairs, or concentrating on a work meeting can feel extra draining. Over time, this can lead to a habit of avoiding physical activity. The less active you are, the more your muscles might tighten or weaken, which in turn can increase aches.

## Health Risks

Long-term lack of rest can raise the risk of problems such as high blood pressure, issues with blood sugar control, and lowered immune function. Poor sleep might also influence appetite regulation, making it easier to gain unwanted weight or crave foods that are not very nutritious.

---

# Strategies to Improve Sleep Quality

## 1. Setting Up a Helpful Environment

- **Cool Temperature**: Night sweats and hot flashes can be reduced by keeping the bedroom at a comfortable, cooler temperature. A fan or air conditioner can also help move air around.
- **Dark and Quiet**: Light pollution from street lamps or noise from neighbors can keep you awake. Blackout curtains, an eye mask, or earplugs might offer relief.
- **Comfortable Bedding**: Soft, breathable sheets and pajamas made of natural fibers like cotton can lessen nighttime sweating.

## 2. Building a Steady Bedtime Routine

A consistent routine signals your brain that it is time to relax:

- **Regular Schedule**: Go to bed and wake up at the same time daily, even on weekends, if possible.
- **Relaxing Pre-Bed Activities**: Read a calming book (avoid thrillers that might be too stimulating), or listen to gentle music.
- **Avoiding Screens**: The blue light from phones, tablets, or TVs can trick the brain into staying alert. Try to stop screen time at least 30 minutes before bedtime.

### 3. Managing Night Sweats

- **Wear Lightweight Sleepwear**: Avoid thick pajamas or heavy socks at night.
- **Use Moisture-Wicking Sheets**: Specialized bedding can help draw sweat away from the body.
- **Keep Water by the Bed**: A cool sip of water can help if you wake up feeling warm.

### 4. Mild Movement Before Bed

Light stretching can loosen tight muscles and lower stress levels:

- **Gentle Neck Rolls**: Slowly roll your head in a circle to release tension in the neck and shoulders.
- **Easy Upper Body Stretch**: Stand and reach your arms above your head, then gently lower them. Repeat a few times.
- **Short Walk**: Some people find that a 10- to 15-minute walk after dinner helps burn off nervous energy.

---

## Lifestyle Adjustments for Better Sleep

### 1. Watch Caffeine and Alcohol

- **Caffeine**: Found in coffee, tea, chocolate, and certain sodas. Consuming it too late in the day can keep you awake. Many people benefit by cutting off caffeine by early afternoon.
- **Alcohol**: It may initially help you relax, but as it metabolizes, it can disrupt your sleep later in the night.

### 2. Mind Your Evening Meals

Large or heavy meals close to bedtime may cause indigestion or heartburn, interrupting sleep. Consider lighter dinners with balanced nutrients. If you get hungry before bed, a small snack like a piece of fruit or a handful of nuts may be okay, but avoid spicy or greasy foods.

### 3. Stay Active During the Day

Regular daytime physical activity can help regulate the body's internal clock, making it easier to sleep at night. Light exercise, such as a gentle workout or a short brisk walk, can also reduce stress. However, it is wise not to do heavy workouts too close to bedtime, as this can increase alertness.

### 4. Manage Stress

Given that stress hormones can affect sleep, try relaxation methods (breathing exercises, writing in a journal, or listening to calm audio programs) to reduce tension. If anxious thoughts keep you awake, some people find that listing tomorrow's tasks in a notebook can help the mind let go of worries.

---

## Tools and Techniques for Chronic Insomnia

If trouble sleeping persists and self-care steps do not help, there are more structured approaches:

1. **Cognitive Behavioral Methods for Insomnia (CBT-I)**: A type of therapy that helps change beliefs and habits around sleep. It often focuses on keeping a sleep diary, improving sleep hygiene, and addressing anxious thoughts.
2. **Relaxation and Imagery Exercises**: Audio recordings guide you through calming scenes or ask you to focus on each part of your body, releasing tension along the way.
3. **Light Therapy**: For people whose sleep-wake cycle is off, spending time in bright natural light during the morning can support a healthier circadian rhythm.

### When to Seek Medical Advice

If you notice ongoing insomnia—trouble sleeping for more than a few weeks—or severe daytime sleepiness, it might be time to speak with a health professional. In some cases, conditions like sleep apnea could be a factor, requiring specialized tests or treatments.

# Boosting Daytime Energy

Even if you manage to improve nighttime sleep, you may still deal with low energy at times. Here are ways to boost energy levels during the day:

## 1. Balanced Eating

- **Frequent, Small Meals**: Instead of two or three large meals, consider smaller meals spaced evenly. This can keep blood sugar more stable.
- **Protein with Each Meal**: Protein helps you feel fuller and supports steady energy release. Examples include eggs, lean meats, beans, or nuts.
- **Avoid Sugary Surges**: High-sugar foods or drinks can give a quick burst of energy followed by a crash.

## 2. Short Breaks

If you work at a desk or do focused tasks, pause for a short break every hour or two. This could be standing up to stretch, walking around, or simply resting your eyes. Short breaks can refresh the mind and body, improving productivity.

## 3. Hydration

Mild dehydration can cause fatigue. Keep water nearby and take sips often. If you prefer flavor, add a slice of cucumber or a small amount of fruit juice to water. Remember that sugary drinks can cause energy spikes and drops, so water or lightly flavored seltzer may be better choices.

## 4. Gentle Midday Movement

If you find yourself sleepy after lunch, consider a short walk outdoors or simple stretches at your workspace. Movement raises blood flow, helping you feel more awake. It can also lower muscle tension, which can grow from sitting still too long.

## 5. Consider Iron Levels

Although menopause-related changes do not usually increase iron needs, if you had heavy or erratic periods during perimenopause, you might be low on iron. Low iron can cause tiredness. If you suspect this, talk to a health expert about checking your levels. Iron supplements should only be taken if you have a confirmed deficiency, as too much iron can cause other problems.

## Dealing with Restless Legs or Other Issues

Some women discover an increased occurrence of restless legs syndrome (RLS). This condition leads to an uncomfortable urge to move the legs, typically at night. It can prevent falling asleep or wake a person from rest. Here are tips if you think you have RLS:

1. **Stretch or Massage Before Bed**: Massaging your legs or doing light stretches can calm the muscles.
2. **Limit Caffeine**: Caffeine can aggravate RLS.
3. **Check Iron**: Research shows that low iron stores may worsen RLS, so testing ferritin levels could be helpful.
4. **Talk to a Doctor**: Medication options are available for those with severe cases.

## Balancing Family, Work, and Personal Time

Midlife can bring multiple responsibilities, such as caring for teenagers or supporting older relatives. These tasks can add stress and make it even harder to sleep well. Some suggestions:

- **Share Responsibilities**: If possible, involve family members or community resources to help with caregiving tasks.
- **Set Boundaries**: Try to avoid working or worrying late into the night. Mark a cutoff time for tasks or phone calls.
- **Use Time Wisely**: If you know you often feel drained in the evening, plan demanding tasks earlier in the day and leave simpler tasks for later.

# Non-Medication Sleep Aids

Various items on the market claim to help with sleep, but results can differ:

1. **Herbal Teas**: Chamomile or other mild herbal blends can be soothing before bed. Be aware that some blends contain caffeine from tea leaves—check labels.
2. **Aromatherapy**: Scents like lavender may calm some people. This can be from a diffuser or drops on a pillow.
3. **White Noise Machine**: Masks background sounds that can disturb sleep.
4. **Weighted Blankets**: Some people report that the gentle pressure from a weighted blanket helps them feel more secure, improving relaxation.

If you decide to try an over-the-counter sleep supplement, read labels carefully and talk with a health professional to ensure it is appropriate for you and does not clash with any medication.

---

# Tracking Sleep Patterns

A simple log can reveal helpful insights:

- **Bedtime and Wake Time**: Note when you turn off the lights and when you actually wake up.
- **Awakenings**: Approximate how many times and for how long you wake during the night.
- **Energy Levels**: Rate your daytime energy from 1 to 10.
- **Possible Triggers**: Jot down evening meals, major stress events, or anything else you suspect might influence sleep.

After a few weeks, patterns could become clear, pointing you toward solutions. For example, you might notice that skipping your afternoon coffee leads to fewer nighttime awakenings.

## Special Considerations: Sleep Apnea

While it is more common in men, women can also develop obstructive sleep apnea. Weight changes during menopause can heighten the risk if extra tissue forms around the throat. Signs of sleep apnea include very loud snoring, gasping, or choking during sleep, and feeling extremely tired all day despite apparently sleeping enough hours.

If you suspect sleep apnea, a doctor might recommend a sleep study. Treatment options can include wearing a device like a CPAP (Continuous Positive Airway Pressure) mask at night to keep airways open. Though this may seem inconvenient, it can greatly improve sleep quality and reduce health risks like high blood pressure.

---

## Tips for Handling Travel or Irregular Schedules

Travel, especially across time zones, can make sleep troubles worse. Here are ways to adapt:

1. **Adjust Gradually**: If flying across multiple zones, try to shift your sleep schedule by an hour or two in the days before you leave.
2. **Stay Hydrated**: Airplane cabins can be dehydrating. Drink water and avoid alcohol on flights if possible.
3. **Block Out Light**: Use an eye mask in hotels if the curtains are not sufficient.
4. **Short Naps**: If you need a daytime nap, keep it short—around 20 minutes—to avoid messing up your nighttime sleep.

For those with shift work or irregular schedules, maintaining consistent routines on off-days can reduce the strain on your body's internal clock.

---

## Combining Physical and Emotional Strategies

We have already mentioned that poor sleep can feed into anxiety, low mood, and irritability. At the same time, emotional tension can worsen sleep. This is why a combined approach is often best:

- **Learn Calming Tools**: Set aside time each day to wind down mentally, perhaps with breathing exercises or mild, slow stretching.
- **Seek Therapy if Needed**: If stress or sadness is overwhelming, a professional can guide you to healthy coping methods. Better emotional balance usually leads to improved rest.
- **Physical Activity**: Regular movement can help manage stress hormones, maintain healthy body weight, and tire you out in a good way by bedtime.

## Encouraging Healthy Habits in a Partner or Household

If you share a room with a partner, their habits can also affect your rest:

- **Snoring or Late-Night TV**: Talk openly about solutions, such as a white noise machine, separate earplugs, or muting the TV early.
- **Different Bedtimes**: If your partner sleeps earlier, try to be considerate if you come to bed later (and vice versa). Minimizing noise or light disruptions can help both of you rest well.
- **Family Schedules**: If you have adult children or teenagers at home who stay up late, set household rules about noise levels after certain hours.

Sometimes, separate sleep arrangements become necessary for a period, such as sleeping in another room, especially if one person's snoring or restlessness keeps the other from sleeping. It is not always ideal, but it can be a temporary way to ensure both parties get enough rest.

## Keeping Expectations Realistic

It is normal to have some changes in sleep as you age, and menopause can amplify those changes. You might not sleep like you did in your early 20s. Instead of aiming for perfect sleep every night, focus on progress—fewer awakenings, feeling better rested overall, or finding methods that help you cope when you do wake up. Self-compassion is important. Blaming yourself or feeling hopeless can raise stress, which can then worsen insomnia.

## Conclusion

Sleep and energy levels often shift during menopause. Hormonal changes, stress, and physical discomfort can combine to disrupt a woman's rest, and this can cause daytime fatigue. However, many strategies are available—from adjusting bedtime habits and staying physically active, to exploring relaxation methods and tracking sleep patterns. Sometimes professional help is needed if insomnia or fatigue becomes severe, or if conditions like sleep apnea are present.

By identifying personal triggers and making small, steady changes, many women regain a healthier sleep pattern and improved energy levels. This in turn supports better mood, focus, and overall well-being. In the next chapter, we will look closely at weight changes and body shape shifts during menopause, and how to manage them with simple, direct methods.

# Chapter 8: Weight and Body Shape Changes

For many women, menopause brings noticeable shifts in weight, particularly around the midsection. Clothing might feel tighter, and the body's shape can look different even if the scale does not show a large change. This chapter explores the reasons behind these weight and shape changes, outlines common challenges, and suggests practical ways to maintain a healthy range that supports overall well-being. We will also discuss less common but important factors such as changes in muscle mass and the role of certain nutrients.

## Why Body Weight and Shape Often Shift

### Hormone Fluctuations

As estrogen levels decrease, the distribution of fat in the body often changes. Before menopause, many women carry fat more in the hips and thighs. After menopause, fat tends to settle in the abdominal area. This can mean a rounder belly or a "thicker" waistline. This is partly due to how cells respond to estrogen and partly because of changes in the way the body breaks down nutrients.

### Metabolism Slows

Most people experience a drop in metabolic rate as they age. The body does not burn calories as quickly as it once did, even with the same eating habits. This slowdown can be linked to:

1. **Loss of Muscle Mass**: Muscle is more active than fat in burning calories. Losing muscle with age means the body uses fewer calories at rest.
2. **Activity Levels**: If aches, fatigue, or busy schedules reduce how much you move, you will burn fewer calories.
3. **Hormones**: Lower levels of certain hormones can change how efficiently the body uses energy.

### Changes in Daily Routines

Menopause often hits in midlife, when many women have work responsibilities, family duties, or other stressors. Skipping regular meals, relying on quick snacks, or forgetting to exercise can contribute to weight gain over time. This is made more difficult if stress leads to emotional eating or if frequent tiredness lowers the desire to cook healthy foods.

## Health Implications of Extra Belly Fat

Carrying more fat around the abdomen is not only about appearance. Research shows that a higher waist circumference can raise the risk of certain health concerns:

- **Heart Issues**: Abdominal fat is often linked with higher blood pressure and cholesterol problems.
- **Blood Sugar Problems**: Too much belly fat can affect how the body handles insulin, increasing the risk of raised blood sugar and possibly type 2 diabetes.
- **Inflammation**: Fat around the waist may produce certain substances that promote inflammation in the body, affecting overall health.

Knowing these risks can motivate a woman to keep an eye on waist measurements and body composition, not just the number on the scale.

## Setting Realistic Goals

Weight control during menopause is usually about health rather than chasing a specific number on the scale. It may not be realistic—or healthy—to aim for the exact figure you had in your 20s. Instead, focus on:

- **A Healthy Range**: A weight range where you feel good and can move around comfortably.
- **Steady Progress**: Small, lasting changes in eating and activity are more likely to stick than extreme dieting.
- **Non-Scale Victories**: More energy, stronger muscles, or improved mood can matter more than a specific weight.

# Practical Dietary Adjustments

## 1. Balancing Macronutrients

- **Protein**: Helps maintain muscle mass, which is key for keeping metabolism steady. Consider lean meats, beans, eggs, dairy, or nuts.
- **Complex Carbohydrates**: Whole grains, vegetables, and fruits provide fiber and steady energy. Refined carbs (white bread, sugary cereals) can spike blood sugar.
- **Healthy Fats**: Avocados, olive oil, nuts, and seeds can keep you satisfied. Trans fats or too many saturated fats can raise health risks.

## 2. Portion Control

What seemed like a normal portion in your 30s may be too large in your 50s if your body is burning fewer calories. Using smaller plates, measuring out servings, or learning to eat until you are about 80% full can help reduce overeating. Eating slowly and savoring each bite allows your stomach and brain to register fullness more accurately.

## 3. Increasing Fiber

Foods high in fiber can help with weight management by creating a feeling of fullness without adding too many calories. Aim for:

- **Oats or Whole Wheat**: Replace white bread with whole grain bread, refined cereals with oatmeal, and white rice with brown rice.
- **Beans and Lentils**: Great sources of protein and fiber.
- **Vegetables and Fruits**: Vegetables like broccoli, carrots, or spinach offer a lot of nutrients with fewer calories. Fruits like berries or apples contain vitamins and beneficial fibers.

## 4. Limit Sugary Drinks and Snacks

Sugars can lurk in sodas, fruit juices with added sugar, flavored coffee drinks, and packaged snacks. These add up quickly without offering much nutritional value. If you have a sweet craving, consider a piece of fresh fruit or a small square of dark chocolate. If you like flavored drinks, try unsweetened teas or water with slices of citrus or cucumber.

## Importance of Muscle Maintenance

### Why Muscle Mass Matters

Muscles burn more calories at rest than fat does. Losing muscle mass with age can slow metabolism, making weight gain more likely, especially around the waist. To help maintain or rebuild muscle:

- **Add Strength Exercises**: Simple moves like squats, push-ups against a wall, or lifting light weights can help.
- **Stay Active**: Even daily tasks like carrying groceries or climbing stairs can build muscle if done regularly.
- **Check Protein Intake**: Muscles need protein to repair and grow.

### Resistance Training Ideas

If you have not tried resistance training before, start gently:

1. **Body Weight Movements**: Squats using a chair for support, modified push-ups on your knees, or planks with your hands on a table.
2. **Light Weights**: Try lifting 1- to 5-pound dumbbells or use resistance bands. Over time, you can increase the weight.
3. **Core Exercises**: Building strong abdominal and lower back muscles supports posture and can help reduce the feeling of a protruding belly, though spot-reducing fat in one area is not possible.

## Physical Activity for Managing Weight

### 1. Cardiovascular Exercise

Cardio activities raise the heart rate, helping burn calories:

- **Walking**: A brisk pace for 30 minutes most days can be a good start.
- **Swimming**: Easier on joints, yet it can raise cardiovascular strength.
- **Cycling**: On a stationary bike at home or outdoors if you prefer fresh air.

Aim for at least 150 minutes per week of moderate-intensity cardio, or 75 minutes of more vigorous exercise, based on health recommendations. Split that time into smaller sessions if it works better for your schedule.

## 2. Interval Methods

Some research suggests short bursts of higher-intensity activity mixed with lower-intensity recovery can be very effective for weight management. For instance, walk briskly for 1 minute, then stroll gently for 2 minutes, and repeat this pattern. This approach can be adapted for many activities.

## 3. Incorporating Activity into Daily Life

- **Park Farther Away**: Get extra steps by parking at the far end of the lot.
- **Use Stairs**: Instead of the elevator, climb the stairs when possible.
- **Break Up Sedentary Time**: If you sit at a desk, stand up and stretch every 30 to 60 minutes.

---

# Emotional Eating and Stress

## Recognizing Triggers

Stress, boredom, or emotional ups and downs can prompt snacking, especially on high-calorie comfort foods. Keeping a journal can highlight patterns—times of day, emotional states, or situations when you feel drawn to mindless eating.

## Healthy Coping Methods

- **Alternative Activities**: If you snack when bored, consider taking a short walk, reading a chapter of a book, or doing a quick craft project.
- **Social Support**: Call a friend or join a community group to share concerns rather than turning to food.
- **Mindful Eating**: Focus on the taste, texture, and smell of each bite. Avoid eating while on the phone or watching TV.

# Supplements and Vitamins

While a balanced diet is the main source of nutrients, some supplements might help certain women maintain a healthier weight:

- **Calcium and Vitamin D**: Important for bones, but may also aid in weight control by supporting metabolic health.
- **Omega-3 Fatty Acids**: Found in fish oil or flaxseed supplements, these might reduce inflammation that can lead to weight gain.
- **B Vitamins**: Support energy metabolism. If you have a deficiency, addressing it can help with overall energy and activity levels.

It is wise to check with a health professional before starting any supplement, as they can advise on dosage and safety.

---

# Monitoring Progress

### Using a Tape Measure

Sometimes the scale does not move much, but the waist measurement decreases. Checking your waist once a month (above the hip bones and around the belly button) can show progress if belly fat is going down.

### Clothing Fit

Noticing a pair of pants feeling looser can be a more encouraging sign than numbers on a scale. Muscle is heavier than fat but takes up less space, so building muscle while losing fat may lead to changes in how clothes fit, even if the scale remains stable.

### Keeping a Journal

A food and activity journal can show you patterns:

- **Daily Meals**: Write down what you eat, including portion sizes and any snacks.
- **Feelings and Mood**: Note how you felt before or after eating. This might help spot emotional eating habits.

- **Exercise Sessions**: Record what kind of activity you did and how you felt afterward.

## Considering Medical or Professional Support

If weight gain is significant or if belly fat is affecting health, consider seeking professional help:

1. **Nutrition Experts**: A registered dietitian can design an eating plan that fits your lifestyle.
2. **Fitness Trainers**: Can create a routine that respects menopause-related changes, joint considerations, and energy levels.
3. **Endocrinologists**: These doctors specialize in hormone issues. If you suspect thyroid or other hormonal imbalances, they can run tests.
4. **Mental Health Professionals**: If stress or anxiety leads to emotional eating, therapy can give new tools for coping.

## Meal Planning Tips for Busy Schedules

### Quick Breakfasts

- **Overnight Oats**: Oats soaked in milk or a milk alternative, with fruits or seeds. Ready to eat in the morning.
- **Hard-Boiled Eggs and Whole Grain Toast**: Quick protein and complex carbs.
- **Smoothies**: Blend yogurt or a dairy-free alternative with berries, spinach, and a bit of nut butter.

### Packed Lunches

- **Salad Jars**: Layer sturdy veggies at the bottom, then proteins like beans, chicken, or tuna, and top with lettuce. Add dressing just before eating.
- **Leftover Grains**: Brown rice or quinoa combined with veggies and a protein can be reheated or eaten at room temperature.
- **Wraps**: Use a whole wheat wrap with lean meats, chopped veggies, and a light spread.

### Easy Dinners

- **One-Pan Roasts**: Place chicken or fish with veggies on a tray, season, and bake.
- **Stir-Fries**: Quick-cooking veggies with lean protein in a simple sauce served over brown rice.
- **Soups or Stews**: Make a larger batch on weekends and freeze portions for a fast weeknight meal.

Planning meals in advance reduces the temptation to grab fast food or high-calorie takeout when tired.

---

# Hormone Therapy and Weight

Some women look into hormone therapy to ease menopause signs. While hormone therapy can help with hot flashes and other problems, its direct effect on weight is less clear. Some women report small changes, but it is not a guaranteed weight-loss method. Instead, talk with a doctor about whether hormone therapy is suitable based on your personal health needs. Focus on maintaining a consistent approach to diet, exercise, and stress management, which are more reliable for weight control.

---

# Handling Plateaus

It is normal to hit periods where weight loss slows or stops. Bodies adapt, and the same routine that worked before may not produce the same results forever. If this happens, consider:

- **Changing Your Exercise Routine**: Increase the intensity or length of workouts slightly, or switch activities to challenge different muscles.
- **Rechecking Eating Habits**: Portion sizes can creep up over time, or mindless snacking might return. A brief food diary might help refocus.
- **Adding More Movement**: If you were doing 30 minutes of walking, try 40 minutes or add a second short walk later in the day.

## Social and Cultural Factors

Friends and family might influence eating patterns. If loved ones prefer big meals or keep sugary snacks in the house, it can be hard to stick to healthier choices. Consider:

- **Open Communication**: Explain your goals. Ask for support or at least understanding about not pressuring you to eat certain foods.
- **Suggest New Recipes**: Instead of avoiding social meals, offer to cook or bring a dish that aligns with your meal plan.
- **Avoid Shame**: Do not feel guilty if you indulge once in a while. A balanced mindset allows occasional treats.

---

## Building a Positive Body Image

Body shape can shift during menopause, and this might affect confidence. It is helpful to remember that healthy living is about feeling good, not chasing perfection.

- **Focus on Strengths**: This could mean recognizing strong legs that carry you through daily life or appreciating that your arms can lift your grandchildren.
- **Celebrate Non-Scale Success**: Increased stamina, better balance, or improved moods are just as meaningful as a smaller waist measurement.
- **Choose Comfortable Clothes**: Update your wardrobe with items that fit your current shape. Clothes that pinch or squeeze can cause discomfort and self-consciousness.

---

## Combining Efforts for Better Results

Tackling midsection weight can be easier when combining balanced eating, smart exercise, and emotional support. Each aspect plays a role:

1. **Nutrition**: Fuels the body with nutrients while managing calorie intake.
2. **Exercise**: Preserves muscle mass and burns calories, plus it can reduce stress.

3. **Stress Management**: Keeps cortisol levels in check, making it less likely that the body will store fat around the abdomen.
4. **Sleep Quality**: Aids hormone balance and prevents cravings triggered by fatigue.

# Chapter 8 Summary

Menopause often brings changes in weight and body shape, especially around the waist. This can happen due to slowing metabolism, decreased muscle mass, and shifts in how the body stores fat. A healthy approach is to make gradual, lasting adjustments in diet, exercise, and daily routines. Focusing on a balanced meal plan with plenty of protein, fiber, and healthy fats can help maintain a steady weight. Including regular physical activities—both cardio and strength movements—supports muscle mass and overall fitness.

Emotional eating and stress can add challenges, but there are ways to cope, such as journaling, social support, or professional guidance. Remember that the goal is long-term health and comfort, not chasing a perfect number on the scale. Keeping realistic objectives, celebrating improvements in strength or stamina, and wearing clothes that fit well can boost confidence during this midlife transition.

In the next chapters, we will continue exploring key health areas for women in menopause, including bone strength, sexual health, and heart concerns. Each subject adds another layer of insight, helping you manage menopause with a well-rounded plan.

# Chapter 9: Bone Health and Strength

Menopause brings changes that affect many parts of the body, including the bones. While bones may seem solid and unchanging, they are living tissues that rebuild themselves over time. When hormone levels shift, this natural rebuilding process can slow or become unbalanced, which can weaken bones. This chapter looks at why bone health matters, how menopause affects bones, and steps you can take to keep them as strong as possible.

---

## Why Bone Health Matters

Bones give shape to the body, protect important organs, and provide the frame for muscles to attach. They also store minerals such as calcium and phosphorus. Once a woman reaches menopause, changes in hormone levels can change how bone tissue is formed and broken down. If bones lose too many minerals, they can become thinner, which may lead to higher chances of fractures or breaks. Keeping bones strong helps with daily tasks like walking, climbing stairs, and bending to pick items up.

---

## How Bones Work

### The Cycle of Bone Growth and Breakdown

The body is constantly building new bone and removing old bone through a cycle called remodeling. Special cells called osteoblasts create new bone, while cells called osteoclasts break down old bone. When these processes are in balance, bone strength stays stable. However, when more bone is broken down than formed, bones can become weak. After menopause, the drop in estrogen often speeds up how quickly bone is broken down.

### Peak Bone Mass

Before menopause, most women reach their highest bone mass in their late 20s or early 30s. This is called peak bone mass. From that point on, the body slowly begins to lose bone. With menopause, the rate of bone loss can increase. However, the higher the peak bone mass you built when younger, the better your bones may handle these losses. Even if you did not have a high peak bone mass, there are still ways to slow further weakening.

---

## Estrogen's Role in Bone Strength

Estrogen helps limit how quickly bone is broken down. When the body's estrogen level drops, the cells that remove old bone can work faster than the cells that build new bone. This can lead to a net loss of bone mass. Not everyone experiences the same amount of bone loss. Factors like genetics, overall health, diet, physical activity, and other hormone levels also play a part.

### Rapid Loss After Menopause

Many women notice a faster drop in bone mass during the first few years after menopause. This stage can last around 5 to 10 years, and then the rate of loss usually settles down a bit. Recognizing the potential for rapid bone changes during this window is important because it can guide you to take actions that slow further weakening.

---

## Osteoporosis: What It Is and Why It Matters

### Defining Osteoporosis

Osteoporosis is a condition where bones become so thin and brittle that they can break with minimal impact. People sometimes mix up osteopenia and osteoporosis. Osteopenia is a milder form of bone loss, often considered a warning that you may be on the road to osteoporosis if no actions are taken. Once a person has osteoporosis, a simple slip or minor bump can lead to a fracture, which can be slow to heal.

## Risk Factors

- **Being Female**: Women are at higher risk because they have lower bone mass than men, and menopause speeds up bone loss.
- **Age**: Bone loss becomes more likely with age.
- **Family History**: If parents or siblings have osteoporosis, your risk goes up.
- **Body Frame Size**: Individuals who are very thin or have a small frame may have less overall bone mass to draw on.
- **Lifestyle Factors**: Smoking, drinking too much alcohol, or not getting enough physical activity can raise the risk.
- **Nutrient Gaps**: Low calcium and vitamin D intake can weaken bones.

## Signs and Diagnosis

Unfortunately, osteoporosis is often called a "silent" condition because people might not realize they have it until a fracture occurs. A bone density scan (often called a DXA or DEXA scan) can show if bones are thinning. This test measures how much mineral is in certain bones, such as the hip or spine. If the levels are too low, it signals that action is needed to prevent breaks in the future.

---

# Nutrients for Strong Bones

### 1. Calcium

Calcium is a key mineral that supports bone structure. Women over 50 often need around 1,200 mg of calcium each day, but the exact amount can vary by health status. Common sources include:

- **Dairy Products**: Milk, yogurt, cheese.
- **Leafy Greens**: Kale, collard greens, bok choy (though the body may not absorb as much calcium from some plant foods).
- **Fortified Foods**: Some cereals, breads, or orange juice have added calcium.
- **Supplements**: Calcium supplements can help fill dietary gaps, though it is best to aim for food first.

It is wise to avoid taking very large doses of calcium in one go, since the body can only absorb so much at once. Splitting your intake into smaller amounts throughout the day can improve absorption.

## 2. Vitamin D

Vitamin D helps the body absorb calcium. Without enough vitamin D, even a high-calcium diet may not be as effective. The body produces vitamin D when the skin is exposed to sunlight, but many factors affect this, like time of day, location, season, and skin tone.

- **Natural Sources**: Fatty fish (salmon, mackerel), egg yolks, fortified milk.
- **Sun Exposure**: Short periods of sun exposure might be enough in some areas, but it varies widely.
- **Supplements**: If your vitamin D level is low, a doctor might recommend a supplement. Vitamin D3 (cholecalciferol) is often preferred.

## 3. Protein

Protein supports muscle and bone health. If you do not get enough protein, the body may have trouble maintaining bone and muscle mass. Aim to include lean meats, fish, beans, or nuts in meals, or try low-fat dairy and eggs for additional protein.

## 4. Other Nutrients

- **Magnesium**: Important for bone structure and found in nuts, seeds, leafy greens.
- **Phosphorus**: Partners with calcium to form bone. Common in meat, dairy, and whole grains, but too much phosphorus (especially from processed foods or soft drinks) might affect the calcium balance.
- **Vitamin K**: Found in leafy greens, it is believed to help with bone metabolism.

# Lifestyle Choices That Promote Bone Strength

## Physical Activity

### 1. Weight-Bearing Exercises

Bone-building activities include walking, dancing, tennis, and other exercises where you stand on your feet and your bones carry your weight. These exercises put stress on bones in a good way, nudging them to stay strong. Even brisk walking for 30 minutes a day, five days a week, can help maintain bone mass.

### 2. Muscle-Strengthening Exercises

Lifting light weights or using resistance bands can increase muscle mass, which supports bones. Strong muscles also improve balance, lowering the chance of falls. Exercises like squats or modified push-ups can be done at home without special equipment.

### 3. Balance and Coordination

Activities such as tai chi (a slow-motion martial art) or certain standing exercises can help improve balance. This lowers the risk of falls that could lead to fractures in someone with weaker bones. Even standing on one foot for short periods while holding a chair for support can strengthen the muscles that help you stay steady.

## Sunlight and Outdoor Time

As mentioned, sun exposure helps the body produce vitamin D. Spending time outdoors can also encourage regular activity, like gardening or a short walk. Take care not to get sunburned. Depending on your location and skin type, 10 to 15 minutes of direct sunlight a few times a week may help maintain vitamin D levels, but your needs could be higher or lower.

## Avoiding Smoking and Too Much Alcohol

- **Smoking**: Studies show that smoking can speed up bone loss. If you smoke, consider resources to help you quit.
- **Alcohol**: Drinking a large amount of alcohol can interfere with bone formation. Keep intake moderate if you consume it.

# Screening and Monitoring

## Bone Density Tests

A bone density test, often done at or after menopause, can help you see if bone loss is happening faster than expected. Your doctor can use these results along with other risk factors to plan possible interventions. Some women with borderline results may have follow-up scans to see if bone density is dropping over time.

## Blood Tests

Doctors may check levels of calcium, vitamin D, parathyroid hormone, and thyroid hormones. Imbalances in these can affect bone health. Thyroid problems, for instance, may raise bone turnover. It is helpful to know if something else beyond menopause is weakening your bones.

# Menopause Hormone Treatments and Bone Health

## Potential Benefits

For some women, hormone-based treatments can slow bone loss by replacing some of the estrogen that the ovaries no longer produce. If a woman has severe hot flashes and is also worried about bone loss, her doctor may suggest hormone therapy. However, these treatments are not for everyone, and possible risks must be considered. In some cases, hormone therapy might protect the spine or hip from losing bone density.

## Other Medical Options

For women at high risk of fractures, doctors might suggest special medications that reduce how quickly bones break down or help rebuild bone. Examples include bisphosphonates, denosumab, or selective estrogen receptor modulators (SERMs). Each has its own potential benefits and side effects, so a doctor can guide you to the best choice.

# Dealing with Fracture Fears

## Preventing Falls

Falls are one of the biggest risks for women with weaker bones. Simple changes at home can lower the likelihood of accidents:

- **Secure Rugs**: Loose rugs can slip around, creating hazards.
- **Good Lighting**: Make sure hallways and staircases have adequate light.
- **Sturdy Footwear**: Shoes with good traction lower the chance of slipping.
- **Organized Spaces**: Clearing clutter from walkways or stairs can reduce tripping.

## Exercises for Stability

Exercises that strengthen the core, legs, and ankles can support better stability. Even using a small step or footstool to practice stepping on and off can build confidence and muscle memory.

## Supportive Devices

If balance is a big worry, a cane or walker can help prevent a fall that might cause a fracture. Though some might resist these aids, they can allow you to remain mobile and independent if used properly.

---

# Life Stages and Bone Health

## Younger Women

If you have daughters or younger relatives, encourage them to build strong bones early by staying active, getting enough calcium and vitamin D, and avoiding smoking. This can help them achieve a higher peak bone mass.

## Post-Menopausal Years

Even after several years past menopause, it is never too late to work on bone health. Exercise and proper nutrition can slow further bone loss. Regular checkups and bone density scans can track progress.

**Long-Term Outlook**

Bone health is a lifelong process. By paying attention to it during menopause, you set the stage for healthier, more active later years. Though you may not be able to stop bone loss entirely, each positive change you make can help reduce the speed at which it happens.

## Common Myths About Menopause and Bone Health

1. **Myth**: "Nothing can be done once bone loss starts."
   **Reality**: It is true that bone loss speeds up after menopause, but many actions—like exercise and proper nutrients—can help slow it down.
2. **Myth**: "Only old people have to worry about fractures."
   **Reality**: Fractures can occur at any adult age if bones are weakened. Early steps can prevent bigger problems later.
3. **Myth**: "High-impact exercise is always bad for bones."
   **Reality**: Some high-impact moves can be beneficial for bone density if done safely. However, people with already weakened bones should speak to a professional to avoid injuries.

## Mental and Emotional Benefits of Strong Bones

Though bone health is mainly about physical strength, it can also affect how a woman feels emotionally. Knowing you are improving or protecting your bone strength can boost confidence in everyday tasks. You may feel more secure walking outside, participating in sports, or simply playing with grandchildren. By reducing worry about fractures, you free yourself to stay socially and physically active, which can benefit mental well-being.

# Detailed Steps to Protect and Boost Bone Strength

1. **Check Your Baseline**: Speak with a doctor to see if a bone density test is recommended.
2. **Optimize Your Diet**: Increase foods rich in calcium and vitamin D. If needed, talk to a health professional about supplements.
3. **Engage in Targeted Activity**: Add weight-bearing activities most days of the week, along with muscle-strengthening a couple of times a week.
4. **Track Your Progress**: Monitor changes in your diet, activity level, or bone density scans. Celebrate improvements such as walking further without fatigue or lifting heavier items more easily.
5. **Seek Help When Needed**: If you have a family history of osteoporosis or experience early menopause, ask a health professional for personalized advice.

---

# Sample Weekly Plan for Bone Health

Below is an example of how a woman might schedule her activities and meals over a week to promote stronger bones. Adjust for your personal preferences and lifestyle:

### Monday

- **Morning**: 20-minute brisk walk outdoors.
- **Lunch**: Salad with spinach, grilled chicken, and shredded cheese.
- **Afternoon**: Light dumbbell routine for arms and shoulders.
- **Dinner**: Baked fish with a side of broccoli. Include a glass of milk or fortified almond milk.

### Tuesday

- **Morning**: Oatmeal with berries; a quick 10-minute round of squats and lunges for muscle strength.
- **Midday**: Spend 15 minutes in the backyard or on a short walk for natural vitamin D.
- **Dinner**: Stir-fry with tofu, veggies, and brown rice.

**Wednesday**

- **Morning**: 30-minute weight-bearing activity like dancing or a walk at a quicker pace.
- **Lunch**: Whole grain wrap with tuna, lettuce, and tomato.
- **Evening**: Check in on how you feel. If stiff, do gentle stretches to keep joints and muscles flexible.

**Thursday**

- **Morning**: Eggs with spinach and a sprinkle of cheese for calcium.
- **Midday**: Gentle balance practice—stand on one foot for 10 seconds, hold a chair if needed, then switch feet.
- **Dinner**: Bean soup with vegetables, plus a side salad.

**Friday**

- **Morning**: 20-minute walk with intervals (2 minutes brisk, 1 minute slow).
- **Lunch**: Yogurt with fruit and a handful of almonds.
- **Afternoon**: Light gardening, if possible, for some physical work and fresh air.

**Saturday**

- **Morning**: If you have time, join a local group walk or low-impact aerobics class.
- **Lunch**: Chicken or turkey sandwich on whole wheat bread.
- **Evening**: Dinner with steamed veggies and a lean protein source.

**Sunday**

- **Rest Day or Leisure Activity**: Could be a gentle bike ride or time with family outdoors.
- **Meal Prep**: Cook in batches for the week, focusing on calcium-rich and nutrient-dense foods.

---

# Overcoming Barriers to Bone Health

- **Time Constraints**: If you are busy, aim for short pockets of exercise spread throughout the day.

- **Budget Concerns**: Canned fish with bones (like sardines), yogurt, or frozen veggies can be cheaper options to boost calcium and nutrition.
- **Physical Limitations**: If you have joint pain or limited mobility, talk with a physical therapist about safe exercises for bone strength. Even chair exercises can be helpful.
- **Lack of Motivation**: Pair up with a friend or family member for walks or workouts. Having a buddy can make the routine more enjoyable.

## Looking Ahead

Bone health is just one piece of a bigger picture in menopause. By giving your bones proper care, you can help avoid fractures and stay mobile. This, in turn, supports an active and independent life. In the next chapter, we will look at another key topic: sexual health and intimacy during menopause. While bone health and sexual well-being might seem different, they both play important roles in a woman's overall comfort and confidence in midlife and beyond.

## Chapter 9 Summary

Bone health becomes particularly important once estrogen levels drop with menopause. The body may lose bone faster than it can be rebuilt, putting a woman at risk for thinning bones and fractures. However, many steps can help:

- Consume Enough Calcium and Vitamin D
- Include Weight-Bearing and Muscle-Strengthening Exercises
- Avoid Excess Smoking or Drinking
- Check Bone Density
- Explore Medical Options When Needed

With practical changes in eating habits, regular movement, and possibly medical support if necessary, women can protect their bone structure and stay strong. This sets the stage for healthier aging, fewer fractures, and increased peace of mind in daily activities.

# Chapter 10: Sexual Health and Intimacy

Menopause can bring shifts in sexual health and intimacy that may feel unexpected or confusing. Some women notice changes in their desire for closeness, while others experience physical challenges like dryness or discomfort. Emotional factors and life stress can also play a role. This chapter explores the ways menopause can affect sexual health and offers tips for communicating with partners, addressing physical problems, and finding new ways to enjoy closeness.

## Why Sexual Health Changes After Menopause

### Hormones and Physical Effects

When estrogen levels drop, certain tissues in the body receive less blood flow and may produce fewer natural fluids. In the private area, the lining can become thinner and less lubricated. This can cause dryness or discomfort during closeness. Lower estrogen may also reduce tissue elasticity, which can make certain movements feel different than they used to.

### Desire and Arousal

Many factors shape a woman's desire, including hormones, general health, emotional connection, and stress levels. With menopause, changes in estrogen and testosterone can influence how easily a woman gets aroused or how strong her interest is. However, it is not always a straightforward drop. Some women notice no decrease in desire, while others see a significant shift.

### Emotional and Lifestyle Elements

Midlife often brings various responsibilities—career, older children, or aging parents—that can add stress and fatigue. Emotional or mental exhaustion can reduce interest in closeness. Also, if a woman feels less confident about her body, that may affect how she approaches sexual activities. Keeping open communication and exploring ways to reduce stress can help maintain a satisfying level of closeness.

# Common Sexual Concerns During Menopause

1. **Vaginal Dryness**: Due to lower estrogen, natural lubrication might lessen, leading to discomfort.
2. **Pain or Discomfort**: Thinner tissues can be more sensitive, causing pain. This might discourage further attempts at intimacy.
3. **Lower Desire**: Some women feel less spontaneous interest in closeness, though they might still enjoy it once they get started.
4. **Difficulty Reaching Pleasure**: Changes in blood flow or sensation can make it harder to reach climax.
5. **Body Image Worries**: Weight changes, hot flashes, or wrinkles can lead to feelings of insecurity.

# Tips for Managing Physical Discomfort

## 1. Moisturizers and Lubricants

Water-based or silicone-based lubricants can help reduce dryness during closeness. Vaginal moisturizers, used regularly (not just before intimacy), can also help hydrate tissues over time. Look for products without harsh perfumes or chemicals.

## 2. Warm-Up and Relaxation

Allow extra time for the body to warm up. Extended foreplay or gentle massage can increase blood flow to sensitive areas, boosting natural lubrication. Relaxation techniques like slow breathing or a warm bath beforehand can also help muscles stay loose.

## 3. Position Changes

Sometimes, using different positions that reduce pressure on sensitive areas can make closeness more comfortable. Experiment with pillows or cushions for support. Talk with a partner to find positions that feel better.

### 4. Localized Estrogen Treatments

If dryness is severe, a doctor might suggest topical estrogen creams, rings, or tablets. These deliver estrogen directly to vaginal tissues with fewer body-wide effects than oral hormone therapy. They can help rebuild the lining and increase natural moisture.

---

## Emotional Aspects of Menopausal Intimacy

### Open Communication with a Partner

Talking about changes is key. If pain or dryness occurs, a partner may not know why you seem less interested. Explaining that hormones are shifting or that certain positions hurt can help both people approach closeness with patience. It might feel awkward at first, but honesty often strengthens emotional bonds.

### Stress, Mood, and Intimacy

High stress can make it hard to focus on closeness. If constant worries about work, family, or finances cloud your mind, it may be difficult to enjoy intimacy. Finding ways to reduce stress—through gentle exercise, brief moments of calm, or counseling—can lift the overall mood and support desire.

### Feeling at Ease with Your Body

Menopause can change the body's shape or lead to dryness, night sweats, or other signs that make a woman feel self-conscious. Building a positive view of your body may take time. Simple steps like wearing comfortable clothing or focusing on what feels good, rather than how you look, can improve confidence.

---

## Low Desire: What to Do

### Is It a Problem?

Desire often fluctuates over life. If low desire does not bother you or your relationship, it might not require any change. But if you feel concerned, or if it affects your bond with a partner, consider exploring causes and possible solutions.

### Rule Out Other Factors

Sometimes, low desire connects to health problems like anemia, thyroid issues, or depression. Certain medicines (for high blood pressure or mood) might also reduce desire. A health professional can check for these. Ensuring your overall health is stable can help with desire.

### Relationship Factors

If there are ongoing conflicts, resentments, or a lack of trust, these can dampen desire. Couples counseling or open conversations may improve emotional closeness. Sometimes, changing how you connect outside of intimate moments—like spending quality time together—can awaken interest.

### Sensual Exploration

Desire might grow if you explore a range of non-intercourse touches. Gentle back rubs, holding hands, or cuddling without any goal in mind can foster closeness. Removing performance pressure and focusing on closeness in smaller steps can help rekindle interest.

---

## Addressing Pain or Burning Feelings

### Communication and Patience

If you notice pain right away, pause and let your partner know. Continuing through pain can create negative associations. Sometimes, a short rest or more lubrication is all that is needed. If discomfort continues, consider scheduling an appointment with a health professional to rule out conditions like infections or thinning tissues.

### Pelvic Floor Exercises

Strengthening the pelvic floor muscles can improve blood flow and reduce some forms of pain. Simple tightening-and-releasing exercises (sometimes known by the brand name "Kegel" exercises) may bring more oxygen to the area. However, if you already have tension in those muscles, you might need a different approach, such as pelvic floor therapy under professional guidance.

## Checking for Infections

If you have itching, unusual discharge, or a burning sensation, you might have a vaginal infection. Menopause can alter the normal balance of bacteria or yeast in the private area, increasing infection risks. A doctor can do tests and prescribe treatments if needed.

---

# Solo Exploration and Self-Care

### Knowing Your Body

Menopause might change how certain touches feel. Some women find that what was once pleasant is now too intense or not enough. Exploring privately can help you understand your body's new responses. This can guide discussions with a partner about what feels good or needs adjusting.

### Stress Relief

Self-care can also reduce stress, which supports a healthier outlook on intimacy. A warm bath, soothing music, or breathing techniques can prepare the mind and body for closeness—whether alone or with a partner. If you struggle with negative thoughts about intimacy, consider journaling or counseling.

---

# The Role of Testosterone

Women produce testosterone in their ovaries and adrenal glands, though in smaller amounts than men. This hormone can affect energy, desire, and mood. After menopause, testosterone levels may also drop or fluctuate. Some doctors explore low-dose testosterone therapy for women who have very low desire that does not respond to other treatments, but this approach is controversial. Side effects, such as unwanted hair growth or mood changes, can happen. If you are curious about it, discussing pros and cons with a well-informed health professional is wise.

# Possible Medical Treatments

If changes in sexual health become distressing, there are medical options:

- **Local Estrogen Products**: As noted, these help with dryness and thinning tissues.
- **Oral Hormone Therapy**: May help overall menopausal signs, including dryness, but it carries possible risks and is not primarily prescribed just for sexual desire problems.
- **Vaginal Laser Treatments**: Some clinics offer laser therapy to help stimulate tissue renewal in the private area. Research is ongoing, and costs may not be covered by insurance.
- **Prescription Medications**: A few medicines target desire issues in women, though they have mixed results and potential side effects.

---

# Psychological and Relationship Support

## Counseling

If tension around closeness builds up, speaking with a therapist can provide relief. Some counselors specialize in sexual concerns. They might give homework assignments or exercises to try at home. If a partner is willing, couples therapy could address problems that hamper closeness.

## Support Groups

Sometimes, hearing how other women handle similar challenges is helpful. Online or in-person groups can reduce isolation. Just remember that each person's body is different, so not every tip will apply. However, listening to diverse experiences can spark helpful ideas and reduce shame.

---

# Rediscovering Fun and Comfort

Sexual health in menopause is not only about preventing pain or dryness; it is also about maintaining enjoyment. This phase can encourage you to look for fresh experiences or ways to connect:

- **Plan Intimate Time**: Busy schedules might leave no room for spontaneity. Setting aside quiet time can help you focus on each other without distractions.
- **Experiment**: Some women find that trying new approaches, like gentle massage oils, new locations, or soft music, can make moments more enjoyable.
- **Focus on the Whole Body**: Closeness is not just about one area. Sensations like gentle stroking of the arms, back, or scalp can be pleasurable.
- **Laugh Together**: If something goes differently than planned, humor can break tension. An open, patient mindset can make closeness feel less pressured.

# Handling Feelings of Loss or Frustration

For some women, the changes in sexual health can lead to sadness, anger, or a sense of loss. It is normal to grieve if you feel an important part of your life is shifting. Let yourself feel these emotions, but remember there are steps you can take to adapt. Friends, therapists, or support groups can offer encouragement and show that you are not alone.

# Body Image and Intimacy

### Accepting Bodily Changes

Menopause can lead to weight gain, wrinkles, or hair thinning, all of which can affect how a woman sees herself. Negative self-image can reduce willingness to be close. Reminding yourself that changes over time are normal and focusing on your positive traits can help. Sometimes, updating your wardrobe to clothes that fit your current shape can boost confidence.

### Partner's View

A loving partner often cares more about the emotional bond than physical details. Open communication about any worries you have can help them reassure you. If your partner has their own worries about aging, discussing these topics together can bring understanding on both sides.

## Exercises to Increase Comfort and Confidence

1. **Pelvic Floor Relaxation**: Lie on your back, knees bent. Take slow breaths, imagining the pelvic area releasing tension. Then gently tighten these muscles for a few seconds and relax. This helps you become aware of muscle control.
2. **Sensory Touch**: Sit somewhere comfortable and slowly run your hands over your arms or legs. Notice how different pressures or speeds feel. This can sharpen sensitivity and guide you in closeness.
3. **Mirror Check**: Standing in front of a mirror might help you become more at ease with the changes you see. This is optional if it feels too uncomfortable, but it can gradually lessen self-consciousness.

## Single Women and Intimacy

Menopause can be challenging for single women as well. They may wonder how to discuss dryness, low desire, or other changes with a new partner. Honesty, when the time is right, is often the best approach. If you plan on dating, remember to protect yourself from sexually transmitted infections—this does not end at midlife. Use protection and consider medical checks if you begin a relationship with a new partner.

## The Social Side of Menopause and Sexuality

Society may send messages that older women are not as interested in closeness, but this is not always true. Many women remain active and satisfied sexually well past menopause. If you face negative stereotypes, remind yourself that personal well-being is more important than societal opinions. Find sources of information that treat older women's sexuality with respect, and consider seeking out supportive communities if you feel judged.

## Possible Questions for Health Professionals

- Is local estrogen therapy right for me?
- Could my medications be affecting desire?
- How can I deal with dryness without hormones?
- Should I consider tests for infections or other medical causes of pain?
- Are there safe ways to address changes in shape or function?

Preparing a list of questions before a medical visit can make it easier to share concerns. Remember that sexual health is a valid topic to discuss, and many doctors are used to helping women find solutions.

## Fostering a Positive Mindset

A shift in sexual health does not mean intimacy must end. Even if some aspects change, closeness can still be pleasant, comforting, and strengthen connections. Keeping a positive outlook, learning new techniques, and staying open to adaptation can enrich your life after menopause.

- **Realistic Expectations**: Understand that some changes are normal, and it may take time to find new comforts.
- **Patient Exploration**: Give yourself permission to explore at your own pace.
- **Communication**: Talking openly with a partner or seeking professional advice can lead to better solutions.

## Chapter 10 Summary

Menopause can affect sexual health in several ways. Lower estrogen may reduce natural lubrication and alter tissue elasticity, leading to dryness or discomfort. Desire can be influenced by hormonal shifts, stress, emotional state, and even body image concerns. Yet, there are many approaches to maintain a satisfying closeness:

- Use Moisturizers and Lubricants
- Consider Local Estrogen or Other Medical Treatments
- Talk Openly with a Partner
- Take Steps to Reduce Stress
- Practice Self-Care

Taking the time to learn what feels right now can lead to deeper emotional connection and physical comfort. Though changes are real, they do not have to mean an end to enjoyment. Rather, they may guide you to discover new ways to experience closeness.

In the upcoming chapters, we will move on to other topics, including heart health, skin changes, and nutrition planning. Each section supports the goal of understanding menopause from many angles, allowing women to adapt in ways that align with their personal needs.

---

# Chapter 11: Heart Health and Circulation

Menopause affects more than just the reproductive system. It can also influence how the heart and blood vessels work. Many women notice that as they age, concerns about heart health come to the front. This is partly because estrogen levels have an impact on blood flow, cholesterol, and other factors. After menopause, the risk of certain heart problems can increase, and staying aware of these changes can help a woman make smart decisions for her well-being.

This chapter covers how menopause can affect the heart and the blood vessels, the possible rise in risk for certain conditions, and what steps can keep the circulatory system strong. We will look at everyday habits, tests that measure heart health, and when to see a health professional. We will also cover less-discussed areas, such as how stress and changes in body shape can contribute to heart issues. By the end, you will have a detailed picture of how menopause can play into heart health and what you can do to protect yourself.

---

## The Importance of Heart Health During Menopause

The heart pumps blood throughout the body, supplying oxygen and nutrients. Blood vessels carry blood to tissues and carry waste products away. When this system works well, we feel energetic. However, changes in age, weight, hormone levels, and other factors can put pressure on the heart and blood vessels.

### Why Risk Might Go Up

Before menopause, many women have a lower risk of serious heart problems compared to men of the same age. Experts suggest that estrogen helps safeguard women's hearts, possibly by maintaining healthier levels of certain blood fats and by aiding in keeping blood vessels flexible. After menopause, estrogen levels drop, meaning that protective effect may be reduced.

In addition, shifts in body weight and muscle mass can affect how the heart works. Gaining extra weight or storing more fat around the waist can increase the load on the heart, while a decline in muscle mass can mean less efficient use of glucose and fats. Also, everyday stress can raise blood pressure, further straining the heart.

# Common Heart and Blood Vessel Concerns

## 1. High Blood Pressure

Blood pressure measures the force of blood pushing against the walls of the arteries. If that pressure stays too high, it can make the heart work harder than normal. Women may notice that blood pressure starts to climb around the menopausal years. Possible reasons include lower estrogen, higher stress, or weight gain. Over time, uncontrolled high blood pressure can damage blood vessels, increasing the likelihood of stroke, kidney problems, and heart problems.

## 2. High Cholesterol

Cholesterol is a fat-like substance in the blood. It is carried in particles known as LDL ("bad" cholesterol) and HDL ("good" cholesterol). Menopause can alter the body's balance of these particles, sometimes raising LDL while lowering HDL. If LDL levels get too high, it can accumulate in the arteries, making them narrower or stiffer. This buildup is called plaque, and it can lead to problems like heart attacks or strokes if it restricts blood flow or forms dangerous clots.

## 3. Atherosclerosis (Hardening of the Arteries)

When plaque builds up over time, the arteries can stiffen or narrow. This process is called atherosclerosis. Early on, a person may not notice any signs. But as it progresses, it can reduce blood flow to the heart muscle or to the brain. Since menopause can accelerate some of these changes, being aware of them is vital.

## 4. Metabolic Issues

Menopause can also influence the body's metabolic processes. For instance, insulin resistance—where cells do not respond as well to insulin—may become more common in midlife. Insulin resistance can raise the risk for type 2 diabetes and also link to higher heart problems. Additionally, weight gain around the abdomen can be part of a pattern called metabolic syndrome, which includes a combination of high blood pressure, high blood sugar, and cholesterol imbalances.

# Signs to Watch For

Heart troubles do not always show obvious signs early on, but there are some warning indicators:

1. **Ongoing Fatigue or Shortness of Breath**: Feeling out of breath during normal tasks might be a hint that the heart is working too hard.
2. **Chest Discomfort**: This can include pressure, tightness, or pain in the middle or left side of the chest. Women sometimes feel pain in the back, neck, or jaw instead of the chest.
3. **Irregular Heartbeat**: A feeling of fluttering, pounding, or skipping beats may or may not be serious, but it is worth checking out if it persists.
4. **Swelling in Legs**: Excess fluid buildup in the ankles or calves can signal circulation problems.

Not all of these signs mean there is a heart condition, but they should not be brushed off. Checking in with a health professional if you notice them often is a good idea.

---

# Steps to Protect Heart Health

### 1. Keep an Eye on Blood Pressure

Aim to have your blood pressure checked regularly, such as once a year, or more often if a doctor recommends it. If you notice readings creeping into higher ranges (above 120/80 mmHg), consider simple changes like reducing salt intake, losing extra weight if suggested, and staying physically active.

### 2. Monitor Cholesterol Levels

A blood test can measure total cholesterol, LDL, HDL, and triglycerides. Based on your results, you can adjust your diet or other habits to keep these values within recommended limits. If numbers are very high, a doctor may suggest medication.

### 3. Move Consistently

Regular activity can lower blood pressure, help control weight, and improve cholesterol levels. Even something as simple as brisk walks most days of the week can have a real benefit. You can also try low-impact aerobics, swimming, or cycling if walking causes joint stress.

### 4. Focus on Balanced Eating

Your meals can directly affect the heart and blood vessels. Foods rich in fiber, such as vegetables, fruits, and whole grains, help regulate both cholesterol and blood sugar. Healthy fats from fish, nuts, and seeds can protect against heart issues. Limiting high-salt, high-sugar, or fried foods can also help keep blood pressure and weight in check.

### 5. Maintain a Healthy Body Weight

Carrying too much weight can strain the heart, but try to avoid extreme diets or drastic changes. A slow, steady approach to weight control typically works best. Keep an eye on your waist measurement, as too many inches around the midsection may indicate higher heart risk.

### 6. Manage Stress

Emotional stress triggers a surge of chemicals like adrenaline and cortisol. Over time, excess stress can raise blood pressure and encourage unhealthy habits (like overeating). Techniques such as slow breathing, short breaks, journaling, or talking to a trusted friend can help. For ongoing stress or anxiety, a counselor or support group may be beneficial.

### 7. Quit Smoking If You Smoke

Smoking damages blood vessel walls and reduces oxygen in the blood, raising heart stress. If you smoke, stopping is one of the most powerful ways to protect your heart. There are many resources and stop-smoking programs that can support this change.

### 8. Moderate Alcohol

Too much alcohol can raise blood pressure, contribute to weight gain, and trigger irregular heartbeats in some people. If you drink, keep it moderate, and be mindful of how it affects your overall health goals.

# Evaluating Hormone Therapy and the Heart

Some women think about hormone therapy (like estrogen or combined estrogen-progesterone) for menopausal signs such as hot flashes. There has been debate over how hormone treatments affect heart health. Earlier studies hinted it might help reduce heart problems if started around the time of menopause, but later research suggests that the outcome varies by individual. It might slightly raise the risk of blood clots, stroke, or certain other issues for some women. This is why it is crucial to talk with a medical expert about your specific risks and benefits.

## Possible Benefits

- May help manage severe menopausal signs.
- Could have a small protective effect on bones.
- For some women, might mildly help certain cholesterol measures.

## Possible Risks

- Raised risk of blood clots in some individuals.
- Potential slight rise in stroke or heart attack risk if started later in life or used for a long period.
- Depends heavily on personal and family medical history.

---

# Tests and Checkups

### 1. Blood Pressure Checks

As mentioned, this is a quick test in most routine medical visits. If you have consistently high readings (130/80 mmHg or higher), your doctor might monitor more closely or prescribe medication.

### 2. Blood Tests

- **Lipid Panel**: Measures total cholesterol, LDL, HDL, and triglycerides.
- **Blood Sugar**: Checking fasting glucose or A1C can reveal if you are at risk for diabetes.

- **C-reactive Protein (CRP)**: Sometimes used to gauge inflammation in the body, which can relate to heart risks.

## 3. Stress Test

If there are concerns about blockages in the arteries or if you have signs like chest discomfort, a stress test can show how the heart handles exercise. It might be done on a treadmill or stationary bike while heart rate and blood pressure are tracked.

## 4. Echocardiogram

An ultrasound of the heart, this test looks at how well the heart pumps, how valves are functioning, and whether the walls of the heart are thickening.

## 5. Coronary Calcium Scan

This scan detects any calcium deposits in the coronary arteries, which can be a sign of plaque buildup. While not used on everyone, it can help doctors assess risk in borderline cases.

---

# Special Topics in Menopausal Heart Health

## Hot Flashes and Heart Risk

Some research suggests that frequent hot flashes, especially early in menopause, might be linked to a higher chance of certain heart problems. Experts are still studying how or why this happens, but it could be related to issues with blood vessel function. If you have very intense or constant hot flashes, it might be worth a discussion with your doctor about overall heart health.

## Palpitations and Irregular Heartbeats

Changes in hormone levels can sometimes cause sensations of a pounding or racing heartbeat. While many cases are harmless, they can feel alarming. If these occur often or come with dizziness, chest pain, or shortness of breath, it is important to get them checked out.

## Variations by Ethnicity

Different ethnic groups may have unique risk patterns for heart-related illness due to genetic, dietary, and social factors. For example, some populations have higher rates of high blood pressure or diabetes. It is good to be aware of any family or cultural patterns that might affect you and discuss them with your doctor.

---

# Putting It All Together in Daily Life

## Balanced Meals

A typical meal plan for heart health might focus on vegetables, lean proteins, whole grains, and limited processed fats or sugars. For example, a day's meals could include:

- **Breakfast**: Oatmeal with fresh berries and a few nuts.
- **Lunch**: A salad with leafy greens, grilled chicken, beans, and a light dressing. Whole grain bread on the side.
- **Snack**: Carrot sticks with hummus or a small handful of almonds.
- **Dinner**: Salmon (rich in omega-3 fatty acids) with steamed vegetables and brown rice.
- **Evening**: A cup of herbal tea instead of a sugary dessert.

## Regular Movement

Aim for about 150 minutes per week of moderate-intensity exercise, such as brisk walking or cycling. If you prefer something low impact, swimming or water aerobics can be gentle on joints. Adding small changes, like taking stairs instead of elevators, can also support circulation and heart function.

## Handling Stressful Days

Menopause can bring added stress from family or work. Setting aside a few minutes of quiet time daily can help lower heart strain. Some women find that journaling worries, doing breathing exercises, or even gardening can bring calm. The key is consistency.

## Social and Emotional Support

Isolation can worsen stress. Try to maintain or build friendships, join community groups, or reach out to family members who support healthy habits. If your circle of friends is small, consider local clubs or online communities focused on healthy living.

## When Heart Problems Arise

If you receive a diagnosis such as high blood pressure, high cholesterol, or early signs of heart disease, do not feel discouraged. Many conditions can be managed through a mix of medicine and lifestyle adjustments. Your doctor may suggest medication to lower blood pressure or cholesterol while encouraging you to keep up healthy habits.

### Medication Tips

- **Take As Directed**: If your doctor prescribes blood pressure pills or statins for cholesterol, follow the instructions closely. Missing doses can reduce effectiveness.
- **Watch for Side Effects**: Report any muscle pains, cough, or dizziness to your healthcare provider. They may adjust the type or dose of medication.
- **Do Not Stop Suddenly**: Quitting certain medications without a doctor's guidance can cause a rebound effect, making the condition worse.

## Overcoming Barriers

### "I Don't Have Time to Exercise"

Short sessions of movement can add up. Try 10 or 15 minutes here and there. Even a brisk walk during your lunch break or marching in place while watching TV can help. If possible, find a friend to join you, as it can make it more enjoyable.

### "Eating Healthy Is Too Expensive"

While certain fresh foods can cost more, there are budget-friendly strategies:

- **Buy Frozen or Seasonal Produce**: It can be just as nutritious.
- **Cook in Batches**: Make large pots of soups or stews packed with veggies and lean protein, then freeze leftovers.
- **Focus on Simple Foods**: Beans, brown rice, and vegetables can form a cheap, healthy base for meals.

## "It's Too Late"

It is never too late to care for your heart. While earlier habits may have taken a toll, each positive change—like improving diet, walking more, or stopping smoking—can show benefits. Blood pressure and cholesterol levels can shift in a matter of weeks to months with healthy changes.

---

# Emotional Well-Being and the Heart

Your mood affects your heart. Anxiety and depression can raise stress hormones, which might harm blood vessels over time. If you struggle with persistent sadness or worry, consider talking to a mental health professional. Counseling, support groups, or low-impact forms of mindfulness can ease emotional strain and, in turn, support a healthier heart.

---

# The Role of Family History

If your close relatives—especially parents or siblings—have a history of heart problems at relatively young ages, your risk may be higher. Share this background with your doctor. They might recommend earlier or more frequent tests, and stricter targets for cholesterol, blood pressure, or blood sugar.

---

# Supporting Others in Heart Health

If you have friends or family members going through similar changes, encourage them to get their blood pressure checked or join a healthy activity. Sometimes doing these things together keeps everyone motivated. Collective cooking of healthy meals, shared walks, and group check-ins can turn a health challenge into a supportive experience for all.

## Summary Tips for a Healthy Heart During Menopause

- **Watch Your Blood Pressure**: Check it regularly, aim for normal ranges.
- **Keep Up with Activity**: Walk, swim, or do something active most days.
- **Balance Nutrition**: Whole grains, lean proteins, fruits, and veggies.
- **Control Stress**: Try short relaxation breaks, stay connected with positive people.
- **Limit Smoking and Alcohol**: Smoking is particularly damaging. If you smoke, find a method to quit.
- **Know Your Numbers**: Cholesterol, fasting glucose, and weight. Regular checkups can spot risks.
- **Consider Hormone Therapy Carefully**: Discuss pros and cons with a professional.
- **Seek Help Early**: If you notice signs of heart trouble, do not put off a medical visit.

## Chapter 11 Conclusion

After menopause, heart health becomes a bigger concern for many women because of dropping estrogen levels, potential weight gain, and other shifts. Monitoring blood pressure, cholesterol, and other risk factors is important. Maintaining consistent exercise, healthy eating habits, and stress management can make a real difference in how you feel and in reducing the chances of long-term heart or blood vessel issues. In many cases, small steps—taken daily—can offer big benefits over time. If challenges do arise, medical approaches and lifestyle adjustments together can help you stay on top of your heart health.

In the next chapter, we will turn to another area affected by menopause: the skin and hair. While they might seem like purely surface concerns, changes in these areas can affect a woman's sense of comfort and confidence. We will explore how hormone shifts impact skin texture and hair growth, plus practical ways to keep both in good shape.

# Chapter 12: Skin and Hair Changes

As menopause unfolds, many women notice changes in their skin and hair. Skin may become drier, less elastic, or more prone to fine lines, while hair can thin or change texture. These shifts are not just about appearance—skin plays a role as a protective barrier, and hair can affect a person's self-image. Understanding the reasons behind these changes helps in taking steps to care for both skin and hair in a realistic, healthy way.

In this chapter, we explore how hormones influence skin and hair, which nutrients can support them, how lifestyle factors play a role, and when to see a professional for stubborn issues. We will also discuss common myths and less common problems, such as sudden hair loss or changes in skin sensitivity. With awareness and the right strategies, women can address these signs of menopause and maintain confidence in their appearance and comfort.

---

## Hormones and the Skin

### The Role of Estrogen

Estrogen helps maintain skin thickness, moisture, and elasticity by promoting collagen production and supporting healthy blood flow. Collagen is a protein that gives skin its firmness and resilience. When estrogen dips during menopause, collagen production can slow. This often leads to drier, thinner skin and the appearance of more noticeable lines.

### Sebum Production

Sebum is the skin's natural oil. It keeps the outer layer soft and offers some protection from dryness. Changes in hormone levels can alter sebum production. Some women find their skin becomes drier; others notice that certain areas remain oily while other patches are dry. This can make picking the right skincare routine more complicated.

### Blood Flow to the Skin

Estrogen also influences how blood flows in small vessels near the skin's surface. With reduced estrogen, blood circulation may decrease, causing the skin to lose some of its glow. When combined with dryness, this can create a dull appearance that feels different from pre-menopause skin.

# Hormones and Hair Changes

## Hair Thinning

Menopause can come with a drop in the hormones that support hair growth. At the same time, the balance of "male" hormones (androgens) to "female" hormones (estrogen, progesterone) may shift. This change sometimes leads to thinning hair on the scalp, though not all women experience it. Hair might lose volume or appear less dense, especially near the forehead or crown.

## Facial Hair

Some women notice new hair growth on the chin or upper lip. This may be related to a relative increase in androgens compared to estrogen. While it can be unwelcome, there are ways to manage or remove these hairs, such as tweezing, waxing, or specialized creams.

## Texture Changes

Hair might become drier, more brittle, or show a different curl pattern than before. Sebum also helps condition the scalp and hair. If sebum production changes, hair might feel rough or less shiny. On the other hand, some women notice less oil, leading them to wash hair less frequently.

# Common Skin Changes During Menopause

1. **Dryness and Itching**: The outer layer may struggle to retain moisture, causing flakiness or itching.
2. **Fine Lines and Wrinkles**: Thinning skin can lead to more visible lines, especially around the eyes and mouth.
3. **Age Spots**: These are small, darker patches that can appear on areas exposed to the sun over many years, such as hands and face.

4. **Sensitivity**: Some women become more prone to irritation from products that never caused problems before.
5. **Slower Healing**: Cuts or scrapes might take longer to mend because of reduced collagen and possibly slower cell turnover.

## Addressing Skin Dryness

### 1. Gentle Cleansers

Switch to mild, fragrance-free products that do not strip the skin of its natural oils. Avoid harsh scrubs or ingredients like sulfates, which can worsen dryness.

### 2. Moisturizing

Use a moisturizer right after bathing to lock in water. Look for products containing ceramides, hyaluronic acid, or glycerin, which help hold moisture. Thick creams or ointments may be more effective than lotions if dryness is severe.

### 3. Lukewarm Showers

Hot water can strip oils from the skin, leading to further dryness. Lukewarm water is kinder. Keep showers or baths shorter, and gently pat the skin dry instead of vigorous rubbing.

### 4. Humidifiers

Running a humidifier in your bedroom can help maintain moisture in the air, reducing dryness in the skin (and hair). This is especially useful during cold or dry weather.

## Minimizing Lines and Wrinkles

### 1. Sun Protection

UV rays speed up the breakdown of collagen. Wear sunscreen with at least SPF 30 daily, even on cloudy days. Hats and sunglasses add extra protection. Reducing sun exposure can prevent further damage and age spots.

## 2. Antioxidant Products

Topical products containing vitamin C or other antioxidants can help fight free radicals and support a more even tone. They might not erase deep lines, but can brighten and improve overall texture over time.

## 3. Retinoids

Over-the-counter retinol or prescription retinoids encourage cell turnover and collagen production. They can help soften fine lines and even out skin tone. However, they may cause irritation at first, so start slowly (once or twice a week) and use a gentle moisturizer.

## 4. Healthy Eating and Hydration

Foods rich in antioxidants—like berries, leafy greens, and nuts—support skin health from the inside. Staying hydrated with sufficient water intake also helps maintain plumpness.

---

# Tending to the Scalp and Hair

## 1. Mild Shampoos and Conditioners

Look for shampoos free from harsh sulfates. Conditioners or hair masks with moisturizing ingredients can help reduce dryness and breakage. Avoid scalding hot water when washing hair.

## 2. Scalp Massage

Gently massaging the scalp with fingertips can increase blood flow to hair follicles, which can support better growth. It also helps spread natural oils along the hair shafts. This might not reverse serious thinning, but can be part of a healthy routine.

## 3. Avoid Overstyling

Heat tools like straighteners or curling irons can make dryness worse. If you must use them, apply a heat-protective spray or serum first. Try to reduce how often you color or bleach hair, as chemicals can weaken strands. If you do color your hair, follow with deep-conditioning treatments.

### 4. Trimming Split Ends

Regular trims—every 6 to 8 weeks—can help keep the hair looking healthier by removing split ends. Split ends can travel up the hair shaft if not cut off, leading to a frizzy or unkempt appearance.

### 5. Nutrients for Hair Health

Protein, iron, zinc, and B vitamins are crucial for normal hair growth. If you do not get enough protein, hair might become weaker. Iron deficiency can also show up as thinning hair. Include lean meats, beans, eggs, or fish in your meals if possible. If you suspect low iron or other deficiencies, talk to a health professional about testing.

---

## Coping with Facial Hair Growth

Facial hair can be surprising or embarrassing for some women, but it is typically normal in menopause. Methods for managing it include:

- **Tweezing or Waxing**: Effective for small areas, though waxing can irritate very sensitive skin.
- **Depilatory Creams**: These dissolve hair at the surface. Test on a small patch of skin first to check for irritation.
- **Threading**: A technique commonly used on eyebrows can also remove lip or chin hair.
- **Laser Hair Removal**: More long-lasting, but usually requires several sessions and can be costly. Works best on darker hair against lighter skin.
- **Electrolysis**: Involves an electric current to destroy hair follicles, leading to permanent removal, but it can be time-intensive.

# Treating Age Spots and Uneven Tone

## 1. Brightening Agents

Products with ingredients like niacinamide, kojic acid, or vitamin C can gradually lighten dark spots. These require consistent use over weeks or months.

## 2. Chemical Peels

A mild chemical peel at a dermatologist's office or medi-spa can help remove the top layer of dead skin, revealing a more uniform tone underneath. However, deeper peels come with more risks and downtime.

## 3. Microdermabrasion

A non-invasive procedure that gently exfoliates the outer layer of the skin. Helps fade minor blemishes and can create a smoother surface. Best used for mild discoloration or roughness.

## 4. Sun Protection (Again)

Age spots worsen with further sun exposure, so always pair treatments with protective measures like sunscreen and hats.

---

# When to See a Professional

### Dermatologist Visits

If you experience severe dryness, rashes, or sudden hair loss (which might indicate an underlying medical condition), it is wise to see a dermatologist. They can check for hormonal imbalances, scalp conditions, or skin disorders that need specific treatment. Chronic itchiness or eczema can also occur around menopause, and a specialist can help manage these issues.

### Trichologist for Hair Concerns

Trichologists specialize in hair and scalp health. They can advise on thinning or breakage, check your scalp for problems like seborrheic dermatitis, and suggest tailored products or treatments. They may also refer you to a doctor if they suspect a deeper medical cause.

## Handling Sudden Hair Loss

While gradual thinning is somewhat common, sudden hair shedding (called telogen effluvium) can happen after major stress, illness, or drastic dietary changes. Hormone swings during menopause can sometimes trigger or worsen this condition. If clumps of hair are falling out or you see more hair than usual on your pillow or brush, talk with a doctor. Lab tests might rule out anemia, thyroid issues, or other triggers.

## Lifestyle Habits for Better Skin and Hair

### Balanced Eating

- **Protein**: Lean meats, beans, eggs, dairy, and fish support both skin and hair.
- **Healthy Fats**: Avocados, nuts, seeds, and olive oil can help maintain skin's lipid barrier.
- **Fruits and Vegetables**: Rich in vitamins A, C, E, and others that promote tissue repair.
- **Limit Sugar and Processed Foods**: High-sugar diets can affect collagen and elasticity.

### Stay Hydrated

Water intake aids circulation and helps nutrients reach the skin and scalp. If you do not like plain water, try adding a slice of cucumber, lemon, or a small handful of berries for flavor.

### Stress Management

Chronic stress can worsen skin conditions like acne, eczema, or psoriasis. It may also trigger hair shedding. Regular movement, breathing exercises, or calming hobbies can help control stress hormones that impact skin and hair health.

## Adequate Sleep

During sleep, the body repairs cells and tissues, including those in the skin and scalp. Lack of rest can lead to a dull complexion and might contribute to hair weakness. Aim for consistent bedtimes and a comfortable sleeping environment.

## Myths About Menopausal Skin and Hair

1. **Myth**: "Washing your face less often prevents dryness."
   **Reality**: Proper cleansing removes debris and helps your skincare products work better. Use mild cleansers, not harsh soaps, and follow with moisturizer.
2. **Myth**: "Gray hair is always coarse and rough."
   **Reality**: Gray hair can feel wiry or coarse in some people, but not in everyone. Regular conditioning can help it look and feel softer.
3. **Myth**: "Only expensive products can help menopausal skin."
   **Reality**: Many affordable options have the same active ingredients. The key is finding a gentle formula that addresses dryness or sensitivity.
4. **Myth**: "Hair thinning means I must be ill."
   **Reality**: Some level of thinning can be a normal part of menopause. If it is extreme or rapid, then a checkup may be needed, but mild thinning is often linked to hormonal changes rather than a serious illness.

## Protecting Skin Beyond the Face

Menopause-related dryness can affect the whole body, not just the face:

- **Hands**: Often exposed to harsh soaps or the environment, hands can become cracked or chapped. Use a thick cream after washing.
- **Feet**: Heels may get rough or split. Soaking feet and applying a foot cream with urea can help.
- **Neck and Chest**: These areas are prone to sun damage. Using sunscreen and moisturizer here helps maintain an even tone.

## Alternative and Professional Procedures

### Botox or Fillers

Some women choose injections to soften lines or add volume. Though not for everyone, these procedures may help those who feel self-conscious about wrinkles. It is important to find a qualified professional, as there are risks like infection or an unnatural look if done improperly.

### Laser Treatments

Different types of lasers target issues like age spots, redness, or fine lines. The intensity and recovery time vary. While they can yield noticeable improvements, they can also be pricey and require multiple sessions.

### Hair Restoration Techniques

For severe hair loss, there are methods like platelet-rich plasma (PRP) injections or hair transplants. PRP involves using a patient's own blood platelets, injected into the scalp to stimulate growth. Surgical transplants move healthy follicles from one part of the scalp to another. These are more advanced options, so they require consultation with a specialist.

---

## Emotional Impact of Skin and Hair Changes

Menopause can already be an emotional time due to physical and hormonal shifts. Changes in appearance might lower confidence or lead to frustration. It can help to remember that these changes are a normal part of growing older and that nearly everyone experiences them in some form. Talking openly with friends, or even a counselor, can ease worries about looks. Some find it freeing to let go of past beauty standards and focus on what feels healthy now.

# Practical Self-Care Routines

Below is an example of a day's routine to care for skin and hair during menopause:

**Morning**

- Clean face with a mild, non-foaming cleanser.
- Apply a daytime moisturizer with sunscreen (SPF 30 or above).
- Comb or brush hair gently, and apply a lightweight leave-in conditioner if dryness is an issue.

**Afternoon**

- Stay hydrated. Aim for at least a few cups of water by midday.
- Reapply sunscreen if spending time outdoors.
- If hair feels dry, spritz with water or a hair mist; avoid too many styling products.

**Evening**

- Use a gentle facial cleanser to remove makeup and dirt.
- Apply a retinol or other targeted product if desired, followed by a rich nighttime moisturizer.
- Consider a quick scalp massage before bed.
- Use a hand cream or foot cream. Cover feet with cotton socks if dryness is severe.

**Weekly or As Needed**

- A hair mask or deep conditioner once a week.
- A gentle body exfoliation using a mild scrub or loofah to remove dead skin and let moisturizers absorb better.
- Check for any new spots or changes in moles—monitoring skin for unusual growths is always wise.

---

# Supplements for Skin and Hair

Some women explore supplements like biotin, collagen powders, or specific vitamins. While these can help in cases of deficiency, results vary. It is better to fix problems in the overall diet first. If you suspect nutritional gaps, a doctor or dietitian can guide you. Over-supplementation can lead to other imbalances.

## Special Cases: Skin Disorders That Flare in Menopause

Certain conditions—like psoriasis, eczema, or rosacea—may worsen around menopause due to hormonal and emotional stress. If you have any of these, consult your dermatologist about adjusting treatments or routines. They might recommend changes to skincare products or prescribe certain creams. Managing stress and getting enough rest can help keep flare-ups in check.

## Strategies if You Dislike "Product Overload"

Some women feel overwhelmed by the idea of multiple products. It is okay to keep it simple:

1. **Mild Cleanser**
2. **Moisturizer** suitable for your skin type
3. **Sunscreen** daily
4. A **scalp-friendly shampoo** and **conditioner** that suit your hair's needs

Add specialized items (like serums or masks) only if you want to address certain concerns, and test them one at a time to avoid confusion about which product might cause irritation.

## Practical Hair Styling Approaches

- **Shorter Haircuts**: A shorter style can make thinning hair less obvious. Layers create the illusion of volume.
- **Root Touch-Up Sprays**: These can cover thin spots or greys temporarily.
- **Scarves or Hats**: Some find it fun to accessorize for sun protection or simply as a style choice.

- **Gentle Coloring**: Semi-permanent dyes without harsh chemicals may be gentler on fragile hair.

## Mindset Shifts for Confidence

It may help to redefine what "beauty" means as you move through menopause. Instead of focusing on looking youthful, aim for healthy skin and hair that feel good to you. You might find that a new haircut, a comfortable wardrobe, or different makeup techniques can highlight your features in a way that suits you now. Recognize that confidence often comes from how you feel inside, and that a supportive attitude toward your body can radiate outward more than any single skin or hair product can.

## Chapter 12 Summary

Menopause can bring about various changes in skin and hair, from dryness and thinning to shifts in texture or the appearance of lines. Hormones influence these features more than many realize. However, practical steps—like gentle cleansing, consistent moisturizing, wearing sunscreen, and eating a balanced diet—can go a long way in protecting and improving skin and hair health.

For hair, focusing on mild products, reducing chemical or heat damage, and maintaining a nutrient-rich eating plan can help slow thinning. Sometimes professional help, such as dermatologists or trichologists, is needed for more stubborn concerns. Though these changes can feel challenging or disheartening, they are common parts of menopause. By keeping a realistic mindset, choosing appropriate routines, and seeking help when needed, women can continue to feel good about their appearance as they move through this stage of life.

In the following chapters, we will shift toward nutrition and meal planning, along with other lifestyle factors, to further assist women in staying strong and well throughout menopause and beyond.

# Chapter 13: Nutrition and Meal Planning

Menopause can influence nearly every system in a woman's body, and one area that many overlook is nutrition. The food and drink a woman consumes can affect her mood, bone health, weight, and energy levels. Because the body's needs change during menopause, planning meals carefully can offer benefits like steadier energy, better digestion, and reduced discomfort from symptoms like hot flashes.

In this chapter, we will look at how to choose foods that support health goals during menopause. We will talk about basic nutrients to include, how to build balanced meals, tips for budget-friendly shopping, and methods to handle cravings. We will also address special considerations, such as food sensitivities or vegetarian diets. By the end of this chapter, you will have a clear idea of how daily meals can bolster well-being during this stage of life.

---

## Why Nutrition Matters in Menopause

### Changing Metabolism

As a woman moves through menopause, metabolic rate tends to slow down. That means the body burns fewer calories at rest than before. Some women notice they cannot eat the same meals in the same sizes they did years ago without seeing changes in their waistlines. Paying attention to meal composition can help avoid unplanned weight gain or energy fluctuations.

### Bone and Heart Support

Certain foods can aid bone density and support heart health. This is critical, because the drop in estrogen can increase the likelihood of bone weakening and can also affect circulation. Eating a well-rounded diet ensures the body gets enough calcium, vitamin D, antioxidants, and other nutrients for strong bones and a healthier heart.

## Emotional and Hormonal Balance

Shifting hormones can affect how the brain processes mood signals. Foods that balance blood sugar and supply necessary vitamins may support more stable moods. On the other hand, diets high in sugary or heavily processed foods might lead to mood swings or energy crashes.

## Digestive Comfort

Digestive function can change around menopause, sometimes causing constipation or bloating. Getting more fiber from fruits, vegetables, and whole grains can keep the digestive system running smoothly. Staying hydrated also matters, as does being cautious about foods that cause sensitivity, like dairy or spicy items for some people.

---

# Key Nutrients to Emphasize

## Protein

Protein builds and repairs tissues and helps maintain muscle mass. Because some women lose muscle with age, having enough protein is important. Good sources include:

- **Lean Poultry and Fish**: Chicken, turkey, salmon, cod, trout.
- **Beans and Lentils**: Great for fiber and protein.
- **Eggs**: Provide protein plus essential vitamins and minerals.
- **Nuts and Seeds**: Contain healthy fats and moderate protein.

A rough guideline is to include some protein at each meal or snack. For instance, adding beans to a salad or having an egg with breakfast can help with daily intake.

## Calcium and Vitamin D

Both of these nutrients help maintain bone structure. After menopause, a woman's bones need extra care, so getting these nutrients becomes even more important. Calcium is found in dairy products, leafy greens, fortified plant-based milks, and canned fish with bones (like sardines). Vitamin D is found in fatty fish and fortified foods, and it is also produced by the body when the skin is exposed to sunlight. If you suspect low vitamin D levels, a test can confirm whether a supplement would help.

## Fiber

Fiber supports digestion and keeps blood sugar steadier by slowing how quickly food is absorbed. Whole grains (oats, brown rice, quinoa), fruits, vegetables, beans, and lentils contain plenty of fiber. Aim for gradual increases in fiber intake, as too big a jump at once might lead to gas or bloating. Drinking more water when adding fiber is also helpful.

## Healthy Fats

Not all fats are the same. Replacing some sources of saturated fats (like those in high-fat meats or full-fat dairy) with healthier options can benefit heart health:

- **Avocados**: Packed with monounsaturated fat and vitamins.
- **Seeds (Flax, Chia, Sunflower)**: Contain healthy fats and various minerals.
- **Nuts (Almonds, Walnuts)**: Provide omega-3 fatty acids, especially walnuts.
- **Olive Oil**: Good for cooking at medium heat or as a salad dressing.

## Magnesium and Potassium

These minerals can help with muscle function, blood pressure regulation, and overall well-being. Good sources include bananas, spinach, potatoes, yogurt, beans, seeds, and nuts. Many people do not get enough potassium, so focusing on fruits and veggies helps fill the gap.

---

# Building Balanced Meals

## Plate Method

One simple method for planning meals is to picture the plate divided into sections:

1. **Half the Plate**: Non-starchy vegetables (broccoli, leafy greens, carrots, peppers).
2. **One-Quarter**: Lean proteins (chicken, fish, beans, tofu).
3. **One-Quarter**: Whole grains or starchy vegetables (brown rice, quinoa, sweet potatoes).

Add a small amount of healthy fat, such as olive oil in cooking or a handful of nuts on a salad, and you have a well-rounded meal. This approach keeps portion sizes in check and ensures a variety of nutrients.

## Breakfast Ideas

- **Oatmeal with Berries**: Top plain oats with fresh berries, a spoonful of nuts, and a splash of milk or plant-based milk. Add a little honey or cinnamon for flavor.
- **Egg and Veggie Scramble**: Cook chopped onions, peppers, spinach, or tomatoes, then scramble with one or two eggs. Serve with a slice of whole grain toast.
- **Yogurt Parfait**: Layer plain yogurt, fresh or frozen fruit, and a sprinkle of granola or nuts.

## Lunch Suggestions

- **Whole Wheat Wrap**: Fill with roasted turkey, lettuce, sliced tomatoes, and a thin spread of hummus or avocado.
- **Bean and Veggie Soup**: Combine beans (kidney, pinto, or black), chopped vegetables, and low-sodium broth for a nutritious soup.
- **Salad with Protein**: Use leafy greens as a base, then add grilled chicken or tofu, beans, and a small amount of cheese or nuts for extra flavor.

## Dinner Options

- **Stir-Fry**: Combine lean meat or shrimp with lots of vegetables (broccoli, carrots, bell peppers) in a light sauce. Serve over brown rice or quinoa.
- **Baked Fish**: Season salmon or cod with herbs, bake, and serve with roasted vegetables and a whole grain side.
- **Bean Burritos**: Fill whole grain tortillas with beans, sautéed onions and peppers, and a sprinkle of cheese. Add salsa or plain Greek yogurt for topping.

### Healthy Snacks

- **Apple with Peanut Butter**: Offers fiber, protein, and healthy fat.
- **Carrot Sticks and Hummus**: Crunchy, filling, and nutrient-rich.
- **Low-Fat Cheese Stick**: Provides protein and calcium on the go.
- **Handful of Nuts**: Almonds, cashews, or walnuts can help manage hunger between meals.
- **Fruit Smoothies**: Blend frozen berries, banana, plain yogurt, and a small handful of spinach for an extra nutrient boost.

---

## Hydration and Beverages

Staying hydrated is essential for temperature control, digestion, and many other processes. Even mild dehydration can lead to headaches or tiredness. Water is best, but there are other options:

- **Herbal Teas**: Chamomile or peppermint can be soothing without caffeine.
- **Infused Water**: Add slices of cucumber, lemon, or berries to plain water for flavor.
- **Milk or Plant-Based Milks**: These can provide calcium, vitamin D, and protein, but watch for added sugars.

Try limiting drinks high in sugar, like soda or fruit punch, since they add calories and can disrupt stable blood sugar. Too many caffeinated drinks can also interrupt sleep or worsen hot flashes for some women, so be mindful if that applies to you.

---

## Budget-Friendly Tips

Eating well does not have to break the bank. Here are strategies to keep grocery costs lower:

1. **Buy Seasonal Produce**: Fruits and vegetables in season are often cheaper and fresher.
2. **Choose Store Brands**: Often, the store's own label has a lower price than name brands without compromising on quality.

3. **Cook in Batches**: Making a large batch of soup, chili, or stew can provide meals for multiple days. Freeze portions for quick dinners later on.
4. **Use Frozen Fruits and Vegetables**: They are picked and frozen at their peak, retaining nutrients and costing less at times, especially out of season.
5. **Plan Meals Around Sales**: Look for deals on proteins like chicken breast or lean ground turkey, then build your weekly menu around them.

## Handling Cravings and Emotional Eating

Cravings can strike at any time, especially if hormones are unbalanced or if emotional stress is high. Here are ways to handle them:

1. **Pause**: Before reaching for sweets or salty snacks, take a moment to ask if you are truly hungry or just bored or stressed.
2. **Healthy Swaps**: If you crave sugar, try fruit or a small piece of dark chocolate. If you crave salt, have air-popped popcorn with a little olive oil and herbs instead of chips.
3. **Mindful Eating**: Slow down and savor each bite. This helps the body register fullness and can reduce the urge to overeat.
4. **Regular Meals**: Skipping meals can lead to intense cravings later. Balanced meals at regular times can stabilize blood sugar and mood.

If you find yourself often eating to cope with emotions, seeking support from a counselor or a friend might help break the cycle.

## Special Dietary Considerations

### Vegetarian or Vegan Diets

Many of the principles above apply, but you will need to pay closer attention to nutrients often found in animal products, such as vitamin B12, iron, and zinc. Good sources include:

- **Beans, Lentils, Tofu, Tempeh**: Provide protein, iron, and some B vitamins.
- **Nutritional Yeast**: Often fortified with vitamin B12.

- **Seeds and Nuts**: Supply protein, iron, zinc, and healthy fats.
- **Fortified Plant Milks**: Can offer calcium, vitamin D, and sometimes B12.

## Low-Lactose or Dairy-Free

If dairy is not an option (due to intolerance or choice), calcium and vitamin D should come from other sources:

- **Calcium-Fortified Juices or Plant Milks**
- **Canned Fish with Bones** (if you eat fish)
- **Leafy Greens** (collard greens, kale, bok choy)
- **Tofu made with Calcium Sulfate**

Check labels for vitamin D as well. Some brands fortify non-dairy products with this nutrient.

## Gluten-Free

If you avoid gluten by need or preference, focus on alternatives like brown rice, quinoa, buckwheat, and gluten-free oats (if tolerated). Plenty of vegetables, fruits, beans, and lean proteins are naturally free of gluten.

## Low-Carb or Other Meal Patterns

Some women find they feel better with fewer processed carbs or less sugar. If going low-carb, emphasize non-starchy vegetables, lean proteins, and healthy fats. You do not have to eliminate carbs altogether, but do choose nutrient-rich sources (whole grains, beans) instead of sweets or refined breads.

---

# Eating Out or On the Go

Restaurant meals or quick lunches at work do not have to derail nutrition. Here are a few ideas:

- **Check the Menu Ahead**: Many restaurants post their menus online, allowing you to pick healthier choices in advance.
- **Ask for Changes**: Order dressings or sauces on the side, choose whole grain bread if available, or swap fries for a side salad.

- **Mind Portions**: Restaurant portions can be large. Ask for a half-portion, split a meal with someone, or box up half of it before you start eating.
- **Include Veggies**: Try to incorporate at least one vegetable side dish, such as steamed broccoli or a side salad.

When traveling, pack portable snacks like nuts, dried fruit, or whole grain crackers. This way, you are less tempted by vending machines or fast-food options.

## Meal Planning Steps

1. **Make a Grocery List**: Start by listing what you have at home to avoid buying items you already own. Then list the foods needed for the week's meals and snacks.
2. **Plan for Leftovers**: Cooking once and eating two or three times can save time and money. Roast a chicken for dinner, then use the leftovers in salads or wraps.
3. **Prep Ahead**: Wash and chop produce so it is ready to use. Cook a big batch of grains and store them in the fridge for quick side dishes during the week.
4. **Portion Wisely**: Use smaller containers for lunches, and measure out snacks so you do not eat from large bags or boxes.

## Avoiding Very Restrictive Diets

Some diets encourage drastic cuts in calories or entire food groups. While they may lead to short-term weight loss, they often leave the body lacking essential nutrients. Extreme diets can also increase stress, disrupt normal eating patterns, and sometimes lead to binge eating later on. A more balanced approach usually proves more sustainable and helps maintain muscle mass while supporting bone health and overall well-being.

# Kitchen Tools That Help

- **Slow Cooker or Pressure Cooker**: Excellent for soups, stews, beans, and lean meats.
- **Non-Stick or Cast-Iron Pans**: Reduce the amount of oil needed for cooking.
- **Good Cutting Knives**: Speed up meal prep. Sharp knives make chopping veggies quicker and safer.
- **Food Scale**: Useful if you want to monitor portion sizes.
- **Storage Containers**: Helps with batch cooking and portioning meals for later.

# Handling Taste Changes

Menopause might alter a woman's sense of taste or smell. Some foods might seem more bitter, while others become less appealing. Here are ways to adapt:

- **Try New Herbs or Spices**: If you once used a lot of salt, consider adding flavor with garlic, onion powder, basil, or oregano.
- **Experiment with Cooking Methods**: Roasting vegetables can bring out sweetness, while steaming preserves a lot of nutrients without adding fat.
- **Keep an Open Mind**: Revisit foods you disliked before. Your taste buds might have changed enough that you now enjoy them in different recipes.

# Emotional Links to Food

Food can be a source of comfort, cultural connection, and enjoyment. During menopause, emotional ups and downs might intensify that link. It can help to:

- **Identify Triggers**: If you notice you crave sweets when bored, find a hobby or call a friend instead.
- **Cook with Others**: Preparing meals with family or friends can add a social element and share knowledge of healthy cooking techniques.
- **Practice Balance**: It is okay to have a treat now and then. Depriving yourself entirely often backfires.

# Supplements and Vitamins

While it is best to get nutrients from whole foods, some women might benefit from supplements. For instance, if a blood test shows low vitamin D or iron, or if you avoid certain food groups, a supplement can fill the gap. However, it is wise to speak with a health professional before starting any new supplements, as too much of certain vitamins (like vitamin A or iron) can be harmful.

---

# Sample 3-Day Meal Plan

Below is an example of how you might structure meals. Adjust portion sizes according to your needs:

## Day 1

- **Breakfast**: Oatmeal with a spoonful of peanut butter and sliced banana. Green tea (caffeine optional).
- **Lunch**: Mixed greens salad with tuna, chickpeas, and a small amount of dressing. Whole wheat crackers on the side.
- **Snack**: Apple slices and a thin wedge of cheese.
- **Dinner**: Stir-fry with chicken, bell peppers, onions, carrots, served over brown rice.

## Day 2

- **Breakfast**: Plain Greek yogurt with berries and a sprinkle of granola.
- **Lunch**: Lentil soup with chopped veggies, side of whole wheat bread.
- **Snack**: Handful of walnuts and a small piece of dark chocolate.
- **Dinner**: Baked fish (salmon or cod) seasoned with herbs, roasted broccoli, and quinoa.

## Day 3

- **Breakfast**: Two scrambled eggs with spinach and diced tomatoes, slice of whole wheat toast.
- **Lunch**: Whole grain wrap with hummus, sliced cucumbers, and leftover chicken or beans.
- **Snack**: Low-sugar granola bar or carrot sticks with guacamole.

- **Dinner**: Lean ground turkey chili with beans and chopped vegetables, topped with a small dollop of plain yogurt.

## Summing Up Nutrition Goals

1. **Steady Meals**: Aim for consistent eating times.
2. **Balanced Plates**: Include vegetables, protein, and a smart carbohydrate source.
3. **Moderate Portions**: Watch portion sizes as metabolism slows.
4. **Focus on Nutrients**: Calcium, vitamin D, protein, and fiber are especially important.
5. **Stay Hydrated**: Water and low-sugar drinks help keep the body running smoothly.
6. **Listen to Your Body**: Honor hunger and fullness signals.
7. **Be Flexible**: If you slip, do not give up—just try to make the next meal healthier.

## Conclusion of Chapter 13

Menopause is a phase where the body's nutrient requirements might shift. Planning meals with emphasis on protein, calcium, vitamin D, fiber, and healthier fats can help manage weight, protect bones, and maintain overall well-being. Balancing meals using simple methods, paying attention to portion sizes, and handling cravings in a mindful way can also support stable energy and mood.

You do not need an expensive or overly restrictive diet plan. Instead, focus on balanced eating patterns, sensible portions, and foods that truly satisfy. Small, steady steps with your daily habits can lead to lasting changes. In the next chapter, we will look at the benefits of physical activity and various methods to stay active, helping to reinforce the progress made through better nutrition.

# Chapter 14: Physical Activity and Movement

Just as nutrition plays a key role in supporting the body through menopause, regular movement is also essential. A woman's muscles, bones, heart, and mood can all benefit from consistent physical activity. Because hormones shift during menopause, it is normal to feel tired or demotivated at times, but staying active helps keep the body strong, supports weight management, and can help with mood balance.

In this chapter, we will focus on how to fit different types of movement into daily life, including activities that boost cardiovascular health, build muscle strength, and improve balance. We will also discuss practical suggestions for overcoming common barriers, like joint pain or a busy schedule. You do not have to be a professional athlete to gain the advantages of exercise—every small amount of effort, done regularly, can support well-being.

---

## Why Exercise Matters at This Stage

### Muscle Mass and Metabolism

During menopause, the body may naturally lose muscle. Less muscle can slow metabolism, making it easier to gain weight, especially around the waist. Strength exercises can combat that muscle loss. Even moderate lifting of weights or using resistance bands can help preserve and build muscle tissue.

### Bone Density

Weight-bearing activities—like brisk walking, dancing, or tennis—apply mild stress to the bones, which encourages them to stay strong. This is important, because the drop in estrogen can accelerate bone thinning. Adding short sessions of these activities a few times a week can reduce the likelihood of fractures later on.

## Heart and Circulation

Activities that raise the heart rate improve circulation and help manage blood pressure, cholesterol, and overall heart health. This is vital, as menopause can bring changes that affect the heart and blood vessels.

## Mood and Mental Health

Regular movement can release chemicals in the brain that enhance mood and reduce stress. Exercise can help with anxiety, sadness, and general irritability that sometimes appear alongside hormonal changes.

---

# Types of Exercises

### 1. Aerobic or Cardio

Cardio workouts raise the heart rate and make you breathe more deeply. Examples:

- **Walking**: An accessible way to start. Vary speed or add hills to keep it challenging.
- **Swimming**: Easy on joints but still a great cardio workout.
- **Cycling**: Can be done outdoors or on a stationary bike.
- **Low-Impact Group Classes**: Many community centers offer sessions focused on gentle aerobics.

Recommendations often suggest aiming for 150 minutes per week of moderate-intensity activity. This could be 30 minutes, five days a week. If 30 minutes at once feels too long, break it into two or three shorter sessions.

### 2. Strength or Resistance Training

Such exercises help retain muscle and bone mass. Methods include:

- **Bodyweight Exercises**: Squats, modified push-ups, or lunges.
- **Free Weights**: Dumbbells, kettlebells, or even filled water bottles.
- **Resistance Bands**: Lightweight, portable, and can offer varying levels of resistance.

- **Machines at a Gym**: If you prefer guided movements, machines can help maintain proper form.

Try strength workouts at least two days a week, targeting major muscle groups: legs, arms, core, and back.

## 3. Flexibility and Stretching

Stretching improves range of motion and can reduce stiffness. Options include:

- **Gentle Routines**: Simple stretches for the hamstrings, calves, hips, shoulders, and neck.
- **Light Floor Exercises**: Lying on a mat, carefully pull knees to chest for lower back relief.
- **Static Stretches**: Holding a pose for 20-30 seconds without bouncing.

Stretching after a workout, when muscles are warm, can be more beneficial and less likely to cause injury.

## 4. Balance and Stability

Menopause can bring changes in balance. Exercises that focus on stability can reduce the chance of falls:

- **Standing on One Foot**: Practice near a chair or wall for safety. Start with a few seconds, gradually increase time.
- **Heel-to-Toe Walk**: Walk in a straight line, placing the heel of one foot directly in front of the toes of the other.
- **Gentle Group Classes**: Some classes might focus on slower movements that boost balance.

## 5. Low-Impact Mind-Body Activities

Some forms of movement bring calm while still working the body:

- **Yoga-Like Stretching**: Helps with flexibility, balance, and controlled breathing.
- **Tai Chi**: Involves slow, flowing movements that can aid balance and reduce stress on joints.
- **Water Aerobics**: A gentle way to move the body, especially if joint pain or extra weight makes land exercises challenging.

# Planning a Weekly Routine

Below is a sample schedule to illustrate how you might spread out different exercise types across seven days. Adjust intensity and length to fit your capabilities and doctor's guidance.

- **Monday**: 30-minute brisk walk (cardio) + 10-minute gentle stretching.
- **Tuesday**: Strength routine using bodyweight (push-ups, lunges, planks) for about 20 minutes.
- **Wednesday**: Rest or light activity day (a short walk or relaxed bike ride).
- **Thursday**: Another 30-minute brisk walk or a low-impact aerobics class.
- **Friday**: Strength with light dumbbells focusing on arms, back, and core (20 minutes). Finish with easy stretching.
- **Saturday**: Fun activity like dancing or swimming for 30 minutes.
- **Sunday**: Balance exercises (standing on one foot, heel-to-toe walks) + a short stroll.

In total, this approach provides a mix of cardio, strength, flexibility, and balance. If you feel overly tired on a given day, shorten or slow down the session rather than stopping entirely. Light movement can help circulation and mood without overtaxing the body.

# Starting Safely

## Check with a Professional

If you are new to exercise or have conditions like high blood pressure, arthritis, or any heart concerns, speak with a doctor before beginning a program. They may suggest certain modifications or warn against specific moves.

## Warm Up and Cool Down

Gradually raise your heart rate at the start of a session. March in place or do slow arm circles for a few minutes. At the end, walk slowly for another few minutes and do some light stretching to help muscles relax.

## Progress Slowly

It is natural to feel motivated at first, but doing too much too soon can lead to soreness or injury. If you have not exercised regularly, begin with short sessions (10-15 minutes) of brisk walking or gentle strength moves. Over time, extend or intensify the sessions as you gain endurance.

## Listen to Your Body

During menopause, energy levels can vary from day to day. Some days you might feel ready for a full workout, and other days you only manage a brief walk. Avoid pushing through significant pain, and watch for signs like dizziness or serious discomfort. A bit of muscle soreness is normal, but sharp or lasting pain is not.

---

# Overcoming Common Barriers

## Fatigue or Low Energy

Hormonal changes, night sweats, or trouble sleeping can sap energy. However, mild exercise often reduces fatigue in the long run:

- **Short Sessions**: Try 10 minutes of a low-intensity activity, and if you feel better, do another 10 minutes.
- **Time Your Workouts**: If mornings are tough, try lunch or early evening.
- **Pair with a Friend**: A companion can motivate you on days you feel sluggish.

## Joint Discomfort

Some women have knee or hip pain as they age. High-impact moves can aggravate those joints:

- **Switch to Low Impact**: Swimming, water aerobics, or cycling put less stress on knees and hips.
- **Strengthen Supporting Muscles**: Stronger leg and core muscles can stabilize joints.
- **Use Joint-Friendly Footwear**: Shoes that absorb shock can lessen stress on ankles, knees, and hips.

### Busy Schedules

Fitting workouts into daily tasks can help:

- **Active Breaks**: Stand and move around the office every hour. Climb stairs during a 5-minute break.
- **Combine Activities**: Walk the dog for a brisk workout, or do squats while waiting for food to cook.
- **Plan Ahead**: Mark exercise sessions on a calendar, treating them as important appointments.

### Lack of Motivation

Menopause can affect mood, making it harder to stay motivated. Ideas to keep going:

- **Set Clear Goals**: They might be "Walk 20 minutes a day, 5 days a week" or "Do strength exercises twice a week."
- **Reward Yourself**: Perhaps treat yourself to a relaxing bath, a new book, or a favorite show after consistent workouts.
- **Track Progress**: Use a simple journal or an app. Seeing improvements can inspire you to continue.

---

## Staying Hydrated During Exercise

Hormonal fluctuations can make temperature regulation trickier, so staying hydrated is crucial. Sip water before, during, and after movement sessions. If you sweat a lot, you may need extra fluids. For moderate workouts under an hour, plain water is usually fine. For longer or more intense exercise, you might need something with electrolytes, but watch for added sugars in sports drinks.

---

## Variety to Prevent Boredom or Plateaus

If the same routine day after day feels dull, try mixing it up:

- **Alternate Environments**: Indoor cycling one day, a walk in the park the next.
- **Join Groups**: Community center classes, walking clubs, or online communities can provide social support.
- **Music or Podcasts**: Listening to upbeat tracks or interesting shows can make longer walks or stationary bike rides more engaging.
- **Set Fun Challenges**: Aim to learn a new dance step or try a mild hiking trail.

This variety keeps the body and mind interested, reducing the chance of quitting because you are bored.

---

# Monitoring Progress

## Methods to Track

- **Fitness Logs**: Record details about each session—duration, type, perceived difficulty, and how you felt.
- **Step Counters**: A simple pedometer or phone app can track steps walked per day. Some aim for 8,000 or 10,000 steps, although this can be adjusted to your level.
- **Strength Tests**: Notice if you can lift heavier weights or do more push-ups over time.
- **Clothes Fitting**: Muscles may become more defined, and clothes might feel looser if you are also managing your diet.

## Setting Realistic Goals

Pick goals tied to health and daily function. For example, "I want to climb stairs without getting winded," "I want to reduce back pain," or "I want to lower my blood pressure." These aims can be more motivating and meaningful than just a number on a scale.

## Exercise Gear and Equipment

- **Supportive Shoes**: Especially important for walking or any weight-bearing activities. Look for shoes that fit well and have good cushioning.
- **Comfortable Clothing**: Clothes made from breathable fabrics can help if you are prone to hot flashes. Layers can be handy if your temperature changes quickly.
- **Home Equipment**: Resistance bands, a yoga mat, small dumbbells—none have to be expensive. Even water bottles filled with sand or small bags of rice can work as weights.
- **Gym Membership**: Might be helpful if you prefer treadmill walking, elliptical machines, or group classes. Some gyms offer discounts for older adults.

## Working with Trainers or Classes

If you are unsure how to start, a certified trainer can guide you on form and schedule. Many local fitness centers have group sessions specifically designed for midlife and older adults. Such classes offer social support and ensure you learn proper technique, reducing injury risks. Ask about free trial classes or short-term passes to find a program that fits your comfort level.

## Adaptations for Chronic Conditions

Conditions such as arthritis, diabetes, or osteoporosis can require tailored exercise approaches:

- **Arthritis**: Low-impact moves (swimming, biking) reduce joint stress. Warm-up carefully to lubricate joints.
- **Diabetes**: Regular movement aids blood sugar control, but you may need to monitor glucose levels before and after activity.
- **Osteoporosis**: Weight-bearing exercises are helpful, but be cautious with high-impact moves if bones are very thin. Balance training is key to prevent falls.

- **High Blood Pressure**: Keep moderate intensity to avoid large spikes in blood pressure. Doctor guidance is important.

## Emotional Benefits of Movement

Physical activity can also relieve irritability or low mood. Engaging in group walks can foster social connections, which combat loneliness. Meanwhile, mild exercise can help calm anxiety by redirecting focus to the body's movement rather than racing thoughts. Over time, these benefits can accumulate, supporting a more positive mindset.

## Making Movement Enjoyable

- **Outdoor Settings**: Walking through nature can offer fresh air and a sense of calm.
- **Music and Dance**: Dancing is both a workout and a source of joy.
- **Goal-Oriented Activities**: Training for a charity 5K walk or practicing moves for a dance showcase can give purpose to workouts.
- **Friends and Family**: Exercise can be a time to bond—invite a partner or a child for a walk or try a new activity together.

## Signs of Overexertion

While movement is beneficial, too much or the wrong kind can lead to problems. Watch for:

- **Dizziness or Nausea**: Could mean pushing too hard or not hydrating enough.
- **Unusual Joint Swelling**: Might signal an injury if a knee or ankle suddenly puffs up.
- **Extended Muscle Pain**: A little soreness is okay, but if it persists or worsens days later, cut back or seek advice.
- **Shortness of Breath at Rest**: Occasional breathlessness during a challenging activity is one thing, but if it lingers afterward, see a professional.

Do not ignore warning signals. Rest and recovery are also vital parts of a balanced approach.

## Desk Jobs and Sedentary Lifestyles

If your job involves sitting for long hours, try these tips:

1. **Frequent Micro-Breaks**: Stand, stretch, or walk every hour for a minute or two.
2. **Simple Desk Exercises**: Chair squats, seated leg lifts, shoulder rolls.
3. **Lunchtime Walks**: A brisk 10- to 15-minute walk around the block can re-energize you for the afternoon.
4. **Standing Desk**: If feasible, alternate between standing and sitting. Even an hour a day can help circulation.

## Home Activities That Count

Movement does not have to be formal exercise:

- **Gardening**: Pulling weeds, digging soil, or carrying watering cans can boost heart rate and muscle strength.
- **Housework**: Vigorous cleaning, vacuuming, or scrubbing floors can work up a sweat.
- **Yardwork**: Raking leaves, mowing the lawn (with a push mower), or shoveling snow (if it is safe) can be quite a workout.

## Supportive Environments

Set up areas at home that encourage movement:

- **Clear Space**: Even a small open area to stretch or do band exercises helps.
- **Equipment Storage**: Keep dumbbells or a yoga mat in sight, reminding you to use them.
- **Media**: Consider streaming guided workouts or using DVDs for structured routines.

## Summarizing an Active Plan

1. **Identify Goals**: Do you want improved stamina, stronger bones, or better mood? Let that guide your choices.
2. **Include Variety**: Cardio, strength, balance, and flexibility all play a part.
3. **Be Consistent**: Short sessions most days are better than a big effort once in a while.
4. **Adjust for Menopausal Symptoms**: If hot flashes strike, wear layers and have water nearby. If joint aches flare, pick gentler forms of movement.
5. **Celebrate Milestones**: Recognize when you can walk further, lift heavier, or feel better overall.

## Wrapping Up Chapter 14

Moving the body regularly offers big gains for women going through menopause. Activities that suit your abilities—like walking, dancing, swimming, or light weightlifting—help maintain muscle mass, support heart and bone health, and lift mood. A balanced approach that includes strength, cardio, flexibility, and balance is ideal. Do not be discouraged by fatigue, joint concerns, or a busy life; small sessions here and there can add up to real progress over time.

As you explore different activities, pay attention to how you feel. If something is painful, adjust or try a different exercise. Make movement enjoyable by pairing it with music, nature, or social interactions. Remember to hydrate and allow for rest when needed. By making physical activity a regular part of life, you support a stronger, healthier body that is better equipped to handle the changes of menopause.

In the coming chapters, we will look at hormone therapies, non-medical approaches, and how to manage mood changes and stress. Bringing all these elements together—nutrition, exercise, emotional support—can keep menopause from becoming overwhelming and can help you stay on track for overall health.

# Chapter 15: Evaluating Hormone Therapies

Menopause can bring uncomfortable shifts, such as hot flashes, intense perspiration, mood changes, or sleep problems. Some women find these changes hard to manage with daily adjustments alone. In such cases, hormone therapy may be an option worth thinking about. This chapter explains how hormone therapies function, lists various forms of treatment, covers potential advantages and drawbacks, and shares tips on talking with health experts to choose what might be suitable for individual needs.

Because every woman's body is distinct, there is no single perfect solution. Understanding hormone treatments can help in making well-informed choices, whether you have been experiencing strong hot flashes, dryness, or other signs that reduce comfort. Even if you decide not to use hormones, knowing about them can be helpful when speaking with doctors or comparing different treatments.

---

## What is Hormone Therapy?

Hormone therapy involves taking hormones—mainly estrogen and sometimes progesterone—to compensate for the decline in these substances after menopause. During the reproductive years, the ovaries produce hormones that regulate cycles and influence many body processes. When menopause arrives, these levels go down. In some women, that drop triggers discomfort or more serious health concerns. Hormone therapy aims to address those issues by adding back some of the hormones the body no longer produces in abundance.

### Types of Hormones Involved

1. **Estrogen**: Often considered the primary female hormone, it is responsible for many physical changes in puberty, monthly cycles, and overall health in adult life. After menopause, lower estrogen can lead to hot flashes, dryness in private areas, and changes in bone health.
2. **Progesterone**: Before menopause, this hormone balances the effects of estrogen on the reproductive system. Women who have not had their

uterus removed typically need both estrogen and progesterone in hormone therapy to reduce the risk of certain uterine problems.
3. **Others (Occasionally)**: In some cases, low-dose testosterone or other hormones might be used, but these are less common. Testosterone is more often related to interest in closeness and energy, but it is not a universal component of menopause treatment.

---

## Reasons Women Consider Hormone Therapy

1. **Hot Flashes and Night Sweats**: One of the primary reasons for hormone therapy is to address hot flashes or persistent night sweats. These can disturb sleep and day-to-day comfort.
2. **Vaginal Dryness**: Falling estrogen levels can cause dryness or soreness in private areas, making closeness uncomfortable or painful. Hormone therapy, especially local estrogen, can help restore moisture.
3. **Bone Protection**: Estrogen can protect bone mass. Some women consider hormone therapy to slow bone weakening if they are at risk for thinning bones.
4. **Mood Support**: Though hormone therapy is not typically prescribed solely for mood concerns, some women report feeling more balanced when using it, especially if they experience intense swings linked to hormonal drops.

Hormone therapy is not a guaranteed fix for every sign of menopause. A decision about therapy usually depends on intensity of discomfort, health history, and a woman's personal choice after reviewing benefits and risks with her health professional.

---

## Types of Hormone Therapy

### Systemic Hormone Therapy

Systemic therapy means hormones circulate through the entire body. This can include:

- **Pills**: Often taken daily, these contain estrogen alone or estrogen plus progesterone.
- **Skin Patches**: Hormones are absorbed through the skin when a patch is worn. Some patches are replaced weekly, others more often.
- **Gels or Sprays**: Applied to the skin, these allow hormones to enter the bloodstream gradually.
- **Injections**: Less common for menopause management but used in specific situations.

Systemic therapy can help with whole-body symptoms, such as severe hot flashes or sleep disruptions. It can also support bone density. However, because it circulates widely, there may be an increased risk of certain side effects for women prone to blood clots or other health issues.

## Local (Vaginal) Hormone Therapy

Local therapy delivers hormones directly to specific tissues. Examples include:

- **Creams or Ointments**: Applied inside the private area to reduce dryness and soreness.
- **Vaginal Rings or Tablets**: Placed in the private area, slowly releasing estrogen over time.

Local therapy is particularly helpful for dryness or minor urinary problems related to tissue thinning, without exposing the entire body to high hormone levels. Women who only experience dryness, without major hot flashes, may find local therapy enough for relief.

## Combined or Sequential

Some hormone therapies combine estrogen and progesterone in one product. Others require taking estrogen all the time and adding progesterone for part of the month. This approach can depend on whether a woman is still in early menopause, her personal hormone patterns, or her specific health risks.

---

# Potential Benefits of Hormone Therapy

1. **Relief of Hot Flashes and Sweats**: Estrogen therapy is the most effective known solution for intense hot flashes in many women.

2. **Better Sleep**: If night sweats are reduced, a woman might sleep more soundly, improving daytime energy.
3. **Help with Dryness**: Local or systemic estrogen can maintain moisture and elasticity in private areas, easing discomfort during closeness or everyday movements.
4. **Bone Protection**: Hormone therapy can slow bone weakening, lowering the risk of certain fractures.
5. **Possible Mood Improvements**: Some women report fewer swings in mood or less sadness, though hormone therapy is not always directly prescribed for mental health.

It is worth noting that while these benefits are real for many women, hormone therapy is not mandatory for every situation. Some find that mild hot flashes or dryness can be managed with simpler, non-hormonal remedies. The final decision is personal and should be guided by a doctor's advice.

## Potential Risks and Side Effects

Hormone therapy is not without risks, and these can vary based on health history, age, dosage, and how long therapy is used. Common concerns include:

1. **Blood Clots**: Certain forms of hormone therapy may raise the risk of clots in the legs (deep vein thrombosis) or lungs (pulmonary embolism).
2. **Stroke or Heart Issues**: In older women or those starting therapy many years after menopause began, some studies suggest a slight rise in stroke or heart events.
3. **Breast Changes**: Long-term combined hormone therapy (estrogen plus progesterone) may slightly raise the chance of breast concerns.
4. **Uterine Lining Growth**: Women with a uterus must often take progesterone along with estrogen to reduce the danger of excessive thickening in the uterine lining, which could lead to unwanted cell changes.

These risks can differ significantly among women. Age, health conditions, family history, and lifestyle (such as smoking or activity level) can all play a role. Often, doctors weigh the positives—like bone support and relief from intense hot flashes—against these possible risks to find a balanced choice.

## Who Might Benefit Most

- **Younger Women with Early or Strong Menopausal Signs**: If menopause arrives early (before age 40) or if signs are very strong, hormone therapy might provide better daily function.
- **Women with Low Bone Density**: If a woman is at high risk for fractures and other therapies are not effective or well-tolerated, hormone therapy could help maintain bone strength.
- **Significant Hot Flashes**: Those who deal with extremely frequent or severe hot flashes that impact sleep or mental health.
- **Major Vaginal Dryness**: When local dryness severely affects comfort or closeness, localized estrogen can be quite helpful.

## Who Should Use Extra Caution

- **History of Breast or Uterine Issues**: Women who have had certain cancers, such as breast cancer, often avoid systemic hormone therapy, though local therapy might be safer in some cases.
- **Blood Clotting Disorders**: Hormones can raise the likelihood of clot formation.
- **Unmanaged High Blood Pressure or Heart Disease**: While not an automatic ban, these conditions require close assessment by a doctor.
- **Liver Disease**: Some forms of hormone therapy may strain the liver further.

A thorough medical evaluation is vital to rule out or manage these risks before starting therapy.

## Forms and Methods of Delivery

1. **Pills (Oral)**: Usually taken once a day. They are convenient but pass through the digestive system, meaning the liver processes them. This can affect cholesterol and clotting factors.

2. **Skin Patches**: Placed on the skin and replaced according to instructions (once or twice weekly, depending on the brand). They bypass the liver.
3. **Topical Gels/Creams**: Applied to areas of the skin where absorption is good, like the arm or thigh.
4. **Vaginal Products**: Rings, creams, or tablets used locally for dryness.
5. **Injections**: Less common for menopause. Usually reserved for specific cases.

The best form depends on personal preference, medical history, and which signs are being addressed most urgently.

## Duration of Use

Hormone therapy is often recommended for the shortest time needed to manage signs, typically a few years, particularly when strong hot flashes or dryness are a big problem. Long-term use (beyond 5 to 7 years) can raise the odds of some risks, though new studies suggest that for some women, extended use might be acceptable with careful oversight. No strict rule fits everyone, so doctors tailor recommendations individually. Regular checkups and open conversations about how therapy feels are key to deciding how long to continue.

## Monitoring and Checkups

If you decide on hormone therapy:

1. **Regular Appointments**: Your doctor may want to see you once or twice a year to check on changes, side effects, and overall health.
2. **Breast Exams and Mammograms**: These can catch any concerns early, especially if you are on combined hormone therapy.
3. **Blood Pressure Monitoring**: Hormones can sometimes affect blood pressure, so it is wise to keep an eye on it.
4. **Bone Density Scans**: If bone health is a concern, scans can measure any changes in density over time.

Being proactive with these checks can help you continue therapy safely if you choose to.

## Myths and Misconceptions

1. **"Hormone Therapy is Always Unsafe"**: Research shows that for many women, short-term therapy started near the onset of menopause can be safe and effective if guided by a professional.
2. **"All Hormone Treatments Are the Same"**: Different forms (pill, patch, cream) and varying doses exist, each with unique pros and cons. A one-size-fits-all mindset is not correct.
3. **"It Cures All Menopausal Signs"**: Hormone therapy can help with hot flashes, dryness, and bone health, but it is not guaranteed to fix issues like mood swings or weight changes for every individual.
4. **"Local Estrogen is as Risky as Systemic Estrogen"**: Local estrogen usually has a lower risk profile because it acts mostly on local tissues instead of circulating widely throughout the body.

## Considering a Trial Period

Some women decide to try hormone therapy for a set period—say 3 to 6 months—to see if it eases their main concerns. If improvement is significant, they may choose to stay on it longer. If they see no change or develop side effects, they can stop. Doctors often recommend tapering off rather than quitting suddenly, to avoid sudden return of hot flashes.

## Alternative or Natural Hormones

You might hear about "bioidentical hormones," which are chemically similar to the hormones the human body produces. Some are available by prescription and regulated for quality, while others might come from compounding pharmacies. Certain women report they feel better on these forms, but it is important to remember:

- **"Natural" is not always safer**: Even bioidentical products carry similar risks to standard hormones.

- **Regulation may vary**: Custom-compounded hormones might not undergo the same testing or standardization as FDA-approved versions.
- **Discuss with a Medical Expert**: If you are interested in bioidentical options, talk with a doctor who understands both mainstream and alternative choices to ensure you make a safe decision.

## Tips for Talking with Your Doctor

1. **Prepare Questions**: Write down what you hope to address—hot flashes, dryness, bone health—and your concerns about possible side effects.
2. **Share Health History**: Be open about any past conditions, family history of breast or uterine problems, and any personal risk factors (like smoking).
3. **Clarify Your Goals**: If your main issue is dryness, ask if local therapy might be enough. If bone health is vital, see if hormone therapy is your best option or if other treatments (like bisphosphonates or certain supplements) might help.
4. **Discuss the Form**: Patches vs. pills vs. creams each have pros and cons. A doctor can help you choose what fits your lifestyle.
5. **Plan for Follow-Up**: Ask how soon you should return for a checkup. Make sure you know what signs to watch for or report.

A good partnership with a doctor can help tailor therapy to your individual circumstances.

## Cost and Access

Insurance coverage for hormone therapy can vary. Some plans cover pills more comprehensively than patches or creams, or vice versa. Generics, if available, might be cheaper than brand-name options. If you face high out-of-pocket costs, talk with a pharmacist or your doctor about affordable alternatives. Sometimes changing the type of therapy or brand can cut costs without losing effectiveness.

# Lifestyle to Complement Therapy

Even if hormone therapy is chosen, it is not a magic fix. A healthy lifestyle can amplify its benefits and possibly reduce needed doses:

- **Balanced Eating**: Adequate protein, calcium, and vitamins can help manage weight and support bones.
- **Regular Activity**: Preserves muscle mass, aids the heart, and supports mood.
- **Stress Reduction**: High stress can aggravate menopausal signs. Techniques like simple breathing exercises or pleasant hobbies can lessen the load on the body.
- **Sleep Hygiene**: Keeping a regular sleep schedule and avoiding caffeine late in the day can aid rest.

Combining hormone therapy with these daily habits often yields the best results.

---

# Planning to Stop Hormone Therapy

Many women eventually choose to stop hormone therapy—either because their menopausal signs have lessened or due to changes in personal preference. A few points to consider:

1. **Tapering Off**: Stopping slowly can reduce the return of hot flashes or other problems. A doctor may suggest lowering the dose over weeks or months.
2. **Monitoring Return of Signs**: Some women see mild hot flashes again, but they might not be as severe as before.
3. **Alternative Support**: Tools such as non-hormonal methods or local estrogen might be used if dryness remains a problem.

---

# Case Scenarios (Hypothetical Examples)

- **Case 1**: A 51-year-old woman has severe hot flashes that ruin her sleep. She also struggles with dryness and mild bone thinning. After talking with her doctor, she starts low-dose estrogen plus progesterone in pill form.

She notices improvements in hot flashes within a few weeks. She follows up every six months for blood pressure checks and mammograms.
- **Case 2**: A 58-year-old woman experiences ongoing dryness but no major flashes. She tries a vaginal estrogen cream and finds it relieves soreness. She does not use systemic hormones, as she had a clot in the past. She continues weight-bearing exercise for bone support.
- **Case 3**: A 47-year-old woman with strong family history of breast issues is cautious about systemic hormones. She decides to manage mild flashes with non-hormonal strategies and remains watchful of bone health through calcium, vitamin D, and regular scans.

Though these are fictional, they show different paths women may take based on risks, preferences, and intensity of signs.

## Conclusion: Informed Choices Matter

Hormone therapy can offer considerable relief for many women facing troublesome menopausal signs. It can help reduce hot flashes, dryness, and bone-related issues. However, it is not suited for everyone, and the potential risks must be weighed against the benefits. Personalized factors—age, health status, family history—make a big difference in deciding whether to use these treatments.

Finding a knowledgeable doctor or specialist is crucial. By having an open dialogue, sharing concerns, and staying on top of regular health checks, a woman can make the best decision about hormone therapy. Keep in mind that there are also non-hormonal approaches for those who cannot or prefer not to use hormones. The next chapter explores some of these non-medical strategies that can also bring relief. Combining informed decisions about therapy with healthy daily habits can set the stage for greater comfort and well-being in the menopausal years.

# Chapter 16: Non-Medical Ways to Feel Better

Hormone therapies can help relieve menopause challenges, but they are not the only path. Many women want additional or alternative approaches to stay comfortable and manage signs such as hot flashes, sleep trouble, mood swings, and dryness. This chapter explores various non-medical ways to address these concerns—lifestyle changes, mindfulness techniques, home adjustments, herbal remedies, and more. While none of these approaches promise a total fix, they can often ease symptoms without the potential risks linked to some medical treatments.

As always, different methods work for different people. Some women find relief through small daily adjustments, while others prefer structured programs or counseling. The goal is to create a toolkit of safe and effective options, whether used alone or in combination with other solutions, such as hormone therapy or prescription medicines.

## Lifestyle Changes That Can Help

### 1. Balanced Eating

We have already covered nutrition in an earlier chapter, but let us focus on how it can specifically help with menopause-related issues. A diet rich in whole grains, vegetables, fruits, lean protein, and healthy fats can help:

- **Stabilize Blood Sugar**: Cuts down mood swings and cravings.
- **Manage Weight**: Reduces strain on joints and can minimize hot flashes (as extra weight can sometimes exacerbate them).
- **Support Better Sleep**: Avoiding large, heavy meals late at night may improve rest.
- **Boost Bone Health**: Ensures enough calcium and vitamin D to combat bone weakening.

### 2. Consistent Activity

A regular workout routine helps in many ways:

- **Hot Flash Relief**: Some women note fewer hot flashes when they stay active (though intense exercise can sometimes momentarily trigger warmth for some, overall effects can be positive).
- **Better Mood**: Movement can release chemicals that help with anxious or down feelings.
- **Quality of Rest**: Tiring the body in a healthy way can lead to deeper sleep.

Even short walks or gentle housework can help if you cannot do a structured exercise routine. The key is consistency.

## 3. Stress Management

Since stress can worsen hot flashes and cause poor sleep, controlling stress is vital. Simple techniques include:

- **Breathing Exercises**: Taking slow, deep breaths for a minute or two can calm the nervous system.
- **Calming Pastimes**: Engaging in crafts or listening to soft music can reduce tension.
- **Light Stretch Sessions**: Spending a few minutes stretching in the evening can relax tight muscles and ease the mind.

If you feel chronic worry or sadness, speaking with a mental health professional may help you learn further strategies.

---

# Techniques for Hot Flashes and Sweating

1. **Layer Clothing**: Wear clothes in layers so you can remove one if you start feeling warm. Choose breathable fabrics like cotton or linen.
2. **Adjust Room Temperature**: Keep fans or an air conditioner handy. A lower bedroom temperature can significantly help with night sweats.
3. **Cool Packs**: Some women place a cool pack or damp cloth on the neck or wrists at the start of a hot flash. This can reduce the intensity.
4. **Limit Triggers**: Spicy foods, caffeine, alcohol, or smoking can make flashes worse for certain individuals. Tracking patterns can help you identify personal triggers.

5. **Slow Breathing**: When a hot flash begins, close your eyes (if safe) and take slow, steady breaths. This can help the body relax and moderate the surge of warmth.

---

# Better Sleep Without Medication

Sleep disruptions can be one of the most frustrating parts of menopause. Long-term sleep medication might not be ideal for everyone. Here are some non-medical strategies:

## 1. Good Sleep Habits

- **Regular Schedule**: Go to bed and wake up at the same times each day, even on weekends.
- **Pre-Sleep Routine**: Spend 30 minutes winding down with a calming book, soft music, or gentle stretches.
- **Avoid Bright Screens**: The light from phones or tablets can delay the release of chemicals that help you sleep.
- **Limit Heavy Meals**: Spicy or large dinners close to bedtime can lead to indigestion or night sweats.

## 2. Comfortable Bedroom

- **Cool Environment**: Aim for a slightly cooler temperature. Use breathable bedding, and if night sweats are severe, look for moisture-wicking sheets.
- **Block Excess Light**: Use blinds or curtains. Even small amounts of light can disrupt sleep signals.
- **Soothing Scents**: Some women find mild scents like lavender calming, though it is not proven for everyone.

## 3. Relaxation Practices

- **Muscle Relaxation**: Tense each muscle group one by one and then release. This can help the body settle before bed.
- **Visualization**: Picture a peaceful place or repeat a relaxing phrase in your mind.
- **Journaling**: Writing down worries can sometimes free the mind so you can rest without racing thoughts.

If sleep problems persist for months, consider checking with a doctor to see if there is an underlying cause like sleep apnea or very strong night sweats.

## Emotional Well-Being Without Drugs

Menopausal changes can affect mood, self-confidence, or overall outlook on life. While hormone therapy or antidepressants might be used in some cases, there are also non-medical ways to support mental health:

1. **Social Connections**: Spending time with friends, joining clubs, or volunteering can give a sense of purpose and reduce isolation.
2. **Light Exposure**: Getting some sunlight during the day can assist in regulating mood-related chemicals. Morning walks are a great way to combine movement and sunlight.
3. **Counseling or Talk Therapy**: Sharing thoughts with a trained professional can help sort out concerns related to body changes, family responsibilities, or personal goals.
4. **Mindfulness Exercises**: Paying attention to the present moment with kindness and acceptance can reduce anxious thoughts. Some resources provide short guided audios or classes in this area.

## Herbal and Natural Supplements

A variety of herbal or "natural" remedies are marketed for menopause. While some women find them helpful, scientific evidence is mixed, and quality control can be inconsistent. Here are a few commonly mentioned:

1. **Black Cohosh**: Often taken for hot flashes. Some users see mild relief; others notice no change. There have been questions about possible effects on the liver, so it is wise to consult a doctor before use.
2. **Red Clover**: Contains substances similar to estrogen. Some women try it to reduce hot flashes, though research results vary.
3. **Soy or Isoflavones**: Foods like tofu, soy milk, and edamame contain plant-based estrogen-like compounds. They may help a bit with mild flashes, but large amounts might not be safe for everyone, especially those with certain health issues.

4. **Dong Quai, Evening Primrose Oil, and Others**: Widely sold but lacking strong evidence. Some women experiment and feel improvements; others do not.

Before beginning any herbal product, discuss it with a health professional, especially if you take medicines for blood pressure, diabetes, or other conditions. Interactions can happen. Also, be aware that "natural" does not always mean harmless.

---

# Acupuncture and Massage

- **Acupuncture**: This traditional Chinese approach involves placing small needles at specific points in the body. Some women say it reduces hot flashes or aids relaxation. Others see little impact. Research is not conclusive, but the risk is generally low if done by a licensed practitioner.
- **Massage**: A gentle massage can loosen tense muscles, enhance circulation, and lower stress hormones. While it might not directly remove hot flashes, it can lessen overall tension, which may indirectly help with comfort.

---

# Cool Clothing and Fabrics

Since many women experience temperature swings, wearing clothes made of cotton, bamboo, or moisture-wicking fabrics can help. At night, lightweight pajamas or a breathable gown can reduce night sweats. Some bedding brands market pillows and sheets designed to stay cool. Though they might be somewhat pricier, they can be a worthwhile investment if night sweats are very disruptive.

---

# Hydration and Cooling Drinks

Drinking plenty of water helps with normal temperature control. Keep a water bottle handy, especially if you sense a hot flash coming on. Some women enjoy herbal teas, which can be drunk hot or cold. If caffeine makes flashes worse, consider switching to decaffeinated versions. Adding slices of citrus or cucumber to water can provide a refreshing flavor.

## Pelvic Floor Exercises for Dryness or Discomfort

While dryness is often addressed by local creams or lubricants, pelvic floor exercises (sometimes called Kegels) can also help maintain blood flow and muscle tone in the pelvic region. They involve tightening the muscles used to stop urine flow, holding for a few seconds, then releasing. Doing them regularly can support better circulation and possibly reduce some aspects of dryness. However, women with certain pelvic issues should speak with a physical therapist for guidance.

## Lubricants and Moisturizers

Vaginal dryness can make closeness painful or lead to itching in daily life. Over-the-counter lubricants provide short-term relief during closeness, while moisturizers can be used consistently to maintain hydration. Look for products without harsh chemicals or fragrances. If dryness remains severe, a health professional might suggest low-dose local estrogen or other treatments, but lubricants and moisturizers are easy first steps.

## Home Adjustments

Small changes at home can improve daily comfort:

- **Quiet, Dim Evenings**: Lower lighting and reduce screen use at least 30 minutes before bed to promote relaxation.
- **Fans in Key Spots**: A portable fan in the kitchen, bedroom, or office can quickly relieve warm spells.
- **Organize Wardrobes**: Keep comfortable layers accessible in case you become too warm or too cool.

- **Soft Lighting in the Bathroom**: If you wake at night, bright overhead lights can jolt the senses. A soft night light can help you find your way without fully waking you up.

## Aromatherapy and Calm Environments

Scents such as lavender, chamomile, or citrus may ease tension for some people. Though not scientifically proven for all menopause signs, the act of creating a calm environment with gentle fragrances might improve mood and possibly reduce the severity of hot flashes. Diffusers or essential oils in a bowl of warm water can spread scent in a room. Be careful if you have allergies or sensitivities.

## Support Groups and Shared Experiences

Sometimes, simply talking with others who understand can bring relief. Whether online forums or local meetups, groups allow women to share tips and stories about what helps. Hearing that others have faced similar dryness, hot flashes, or emotional ups and downs can lessen feelings of isolation. You might also gain practical tips like favorite brands of cooling sheets or how someone overcame sleep troubles without medication.

## Partner Communication

For women who have a close relationship, explaining menopausal changes can help a partner understand why you might need a fan on at night, why closeness might feel uncomfortable if dryness is an issue, or why mood swings happen. Calm, honest conversations can prevent misunderstandings and create a supportive environment at home. If dryness makes closeness challenging, consider suggesting extended foreplay or using a lubricant, so both partners can enjoy time together without pain or frustration.

## Non-Drug Support for Mood Changes

1. **Light Therapy**: If low mood is more intense in darker months, a light therapy box could help regulate internal patterns.
2. **Daily Walks**: Gentle sunlight and movement can lift spirits.
3. **Self-Reflection**: Writing down positive events each day—like a short gratitude list—can shift focus to uplifting moments.
4. **Creativity**: Painting, knitting, or learning a simple instrument can channel emotions into new skills.

If mood changes are very intense or prolonged, a counselor, psychologist, or psychiatrist can offer tools and possibly suggest medicines if needed. But many prefer trying non-drug methods initially, especially if mood shifts are mild to moderate.

---

## Mindful Breathing for Hot Flashes

When a hot flash hits, adrenaline can make the heart race. A technique called paced breathing might help. Slowly inhale through the nose for a count of four, hold for a moment, then exhale through the mouth for a count of four. Repeat several times. Some women say it shortens or lessens the discomfort of flashes. If combined with a mental image of a cool place—like imagining a gentle breeze—it can further calm the mind.

---

## Trying New Hobbies

Midlife can be a time of transition. Engaging in new hobbies or revisiting old interests can add excitement and take attention away from menopausal struggles. Whether it is pottery, bird watching, or a cooking class, pursuing fresh activities can deliver a sense of achievement and keep the mind occupied in a positive way.

---

# Tracking Progress

Keeping a simple journal can help you see if certain approaches are making a difference. Note items like:

- **Frequency/Intensity of Hot Flashes**: Did they go down after you began using a cooling pillow at night?
- **Sleep Patterns**: Does no screen time before bed help you sleep longer?
- **Mood**: Did short daily walks improve your sense of calm?

Over a few weeks, patterns might emerge. This can guide you on which strategies to keep and which to skip.

---

# Combining Non-Medical Approaches

Often, the best results come from mixing several methods:

- **Daytime**: Balanced meals, short exercise sessions, simple stress breaks (like slow breathing or journaling).
- **Evening**: A cooler bedroom with a fan and comfortable sheets, plus a gentle stretching routine.
- **General**: Cutting back on triggers like caffeine or spicy foods, using layered clothing, and leaning on social support.

Each method alone might offer a little help, but the total effect can be significant when they are combined.

---

# When Non-Medical Steps Are Not Enough

It is important to acknowledge that some women have very strong menopausal signs that deeply harm daily life. In such cases, speaking with a doctor about medical treatments, including hormone therapy or non-hormonal prescription options, could be worthwhile. Non-medical methods can still be used alongside medical treatments to maximize comfort and lower needed doses of medicines.

# Conclusion: A Toolkit of Healthy Approaches

Non-medical ways to feel better can be very helpful for managing menopause. Adjustments in daily habits, environment, and mindset often make a clear difference, especially when used consistently. While no single trick eliminates all menopausal challenges, combining multiple approaches can bring relief for many women.

Remember to be patient with yourself—some methods may take a few weeks before you notice changes. Also, keep in mind that listening to your body is key. If a certain technique brings frustration or new discomfort, it may not be for you. On the other hand, if something sparks a positive effect, keep it in your routine.

In the next chapters, we will explore further topics such as mood changes and mental health, stress handling, and staying healthy in the long run. Putting together a personalized plan—including non-medical approaches, potential medical treatments, and emotional support—can help you live as comfortably and confidently as possible through the menopausal stage.

# Chapter 17: Mood Changes and Mental Health

Mood changes are common during menopause. A woman might feel more worried, discouraged, or quick to anger. Some feel as though their emotions can shift from calm to tense within minutes. While this can be confusing, there are reasons behind these emotional changes. Hormone drops, sleep problems, and social factors all play a part. The good news is that awareness of these influences, plus some practical steps, can make a difference.

In this chapter, we will explore how menopause affects emotional well-being. We will look at possible causes of mood shifts, ways to address them with daily strategies, and when it might help to see a professional. We will also share ideas on speaking to loved ones about how you feel. By the end of this chapter, you will have a clearer idea of why emotional ups and downs happen and what you can do about them.

---

## How Hormones Affect Emotions

### Changes in Estrogen and Other Hormones

Before menopause, hormones like estrogen and progesterone rise and fall each month, following regular cycles. Once menopause nears, these cycles become unpredictable. Estrogen can drop sharply, then spike, and fall again. Such rapid changes can lead to shifts in the brain chemicals that manage emotion, energy, and focus.

### Effects on Mood Chemicals

For instance, estrogen can influence levels of serotonin and norepinephrine. These substances help regulate feelings of calm or alertness. When estrogen decreases, your levels of certain mood chemicals might dip, leading to feelings like anxiousness or sadness. Not every woman experiences this strongly, but it can be a major factor in emotional ups and downs.

## Sleep Deprivation's Impact on Mood

If you do not rest well due to night sweats or restlessness, your mood can be harder to manage the next day. Poor rest makes the brain less able to handle daily stress. Menopause-related night sweats might wake you multiple times, leading to a shorter or lighter sleep overall. Over time, chronic lack of rest can contribute to low mood or less tolerance for normal daily challenges.

---

## Common Emotional Signs

1. **Mood Swings**: Sudden shifts from content to irritated, worried, or sad.
2. **Feeling Down**: This can range from mild sadness to more pronounced low feelings.
3. **Irritability**: Simple annoyances might feel bigger than usual, leading to more arguments or tensions with family or coworkers.
4. **Anxious Feelings**: Menopause can bring new worries about health, aging, or family roles.
5. **Loss of Motivation**: Some women find they do not enjoy certain activities as much as before or feel less interest in starting new projects.

Not everyone experiences all of these signs, and they can vary in intensity. Some women have short-term issues while others feel them for several years. If these feelings become so strong that they start interfering with life, it may be time to seek help.

---

## Daily Strategies to Support Emotional Balance

### 1. Keeping a Consistent Routine

Having a predictable daily flow can help you feel grounded. Going to bed and getting up at the same time each day keeps your body clock steady, which can help with mood stability. Setting mealtimes and small breaks for yourself at regular intervals can also promote a sense of structure.

### 2. Balanced Nutrition and Hydration

We discussed nutrition in a previous chapter, but here's how it relates to mood:

- **Stable Blood Sugar**: When you skip meals or eat very sugary foods, your blood sugar can swing up and down quickly. This can lead to irritability or difficulty focusing. A balanced meal with protein, whole grains, and veggies keeps blood sugar more level.
- **Hydration**: Mild dehydration can cause fatigue and unclear thinking. Keep a water bottle close by, especially if you are prone to hot flashes.

## 3. Consistent Physical Activity

Moving the body—through walking, dancing, or other low-impact exercises—helps release mood-lifting chemicals. It can also reduce stress hormones. Even small daily movement sessions can make a difference. For example, a 15-minute walk in the neighborhood can clear the mind, boost energy, and lessen restlessness.

## 4. Calming Practices

- **Breathing Exercises**: If you sense a wave of worry or anger, slow, steady breathing can help. Breathe in through the nose for four counts, pause briefly, then exhale through the mouth for four counts.
- **Basic Stretching**: Gentle stretches in the morning or before bed can ease muscle tension and center your thoughts.
- **Quiet Reflection**: Taking five minutes of silence to sit and let thoughts drift can calm a racing mind. Some call this mindfulness, but it can be as simple as pausing to note your thoughts without judging them.

## 5. Staying in Touch with Loved Ones

Isolation or feeling no one understands can make mood swings worse. Sharing your feelings with trusted friends or family can ease tension. You might say, "I'm going through some changes that can affect my mood. I appreciate your patience." A supportive network can remind you that you are not alone.

---

# Recognizing More Severe Mood Problems

Sometimes menopause can coincide with major emotional challenges, such as prolonged low mood or a diagnosed condition like depression or an anxiety disorder. Warning signs:

- **Feelings of Hopelessness**: If you often think that life has no joy or that tasks feel pointless.
- **Loss of Interest**: Activities you once enjoyed bring no pleasure or seem dull.
- **Changes in Appetite or Sleep**: Eating much more or less than usual, or having trouble sleeping most nights.
- **Thoughts of Harm**: If you consider hurting yourself or think life is not worth living. This is a crisis situation that requires immediate help.

In these cases, seeing a mental health professional is vital. Therapy, counseling, or short-term use of certain medicines can help stabilize mood while you go through menopause.

---

# Talking with Health Professionals

### 1. Bring Up Emotional Signs

When visiting a doctor for menopause-related questions, do not hesitate to mention mood changes. Sometimes, doctors focus on hot flashes, dryness, or bone health, but emotional well-being is just as important. They may suggest counseling, refer you to a specialist, or discuss whether certain treatments might help with both physical and emotional signs.

### 2. Medication Options (Non-Hormonal)

Some women benefit from short-term use of medicines typically used for low mood or anxious feelings if symptoms are serious. These might include certain SSRI or SNRI medicines, which can also reduce hot flashes for some. If you already take medication for low mood, your dosage or type of medicine may need adjustment during menopause. Always consult a qualified professional and never stop or start such medications on your own.

### 3. Therapy and Counseling

A counselor or therapist can teach coping methods to handle mood swings. They can also help you see if there are life stressors—beyond just menopause—that might be fueling emotional challenges. Therapy is often a safe space to vent worries without feeling judged.

## Home Environment for Emotional Ease

Since hormone changes can raise tension, setting up a comforting home environment can help:

- **Calming Colors**: Soft blues, greens, or neutrals can make a space feel peaceful.
- **Reduce Clutter**: A cluttered home can add to stress. Having organized areas can lower overwhelm.
- **Soothing Sounds**: Gentle music or nature sounds in the background might help if sudden noises startle or irritate you easily.
- **Personal Space**: If possible, have a quiet corner or room where you can rest or practice breathing exercises when feeling stressed or emotional.

## Managing Relationships During Mood Swings

Menopause can strain relationships if mood changes are severe. You may find yourself snapping at a partner, children, or coworkers for minor reasons. Strategies:

1. **Discuss Triggers**: If certain topics or times of day trigger irritability, mention it to those around you. For example, "I get tense when I first come home from work, so let's talk about tough issues later."
2. **Apologize When Needed**: If you do become short-tempered, a sincere apology can mend hurt feelings. Explain briefly that you are dealing with hormonal shifts.
3. **Problem-Solve Together**: If dryness or low energy affect closeness with a partner, brainstorm solutions. Maybe schedule intimate time when you're feeling calmer or incorporate more gentle approaches that reduce physical discomfort.
4. **Seek Joint Counseling**: If the strain on a relationship is big, meeting with a therapist together can offer tools and new ways of communication.

# Self-Care Ideas for Emotional Well-Being

## 1. Journaling

Writing your thoughts or daily events can help you notice triggers or patterns in mood. Some women keep a brief log of their emotional state, noting if anything special happened that day (like less sleep or more stress) to see what might be at play.

## 2. Creative Outlets

Crafts, painting, music, or simple sketching can direct intense emotions into a more soothing activity. Even if you do not think of yourself as "artistic," these hobbies can reduce worries and provide a sense of achievement.

## 3. Relaxing Hobbies

Gardening, reading, or mild cooking projects can slow the mind and keep hands busy. Hobbies are especially helpful if they do not involve constant phone or internet use, allowing you to step away from potential online stress.

## 4. Gentle Time in Nature

A short walk in a local park or even sitting in a backyard or on a balcony can be refreshing. Observing trees, birds, or open sky can give the brain a rest from daily concerns.

---

# Group Support and Programs

Some communities have programs or gatherings dedicated to women in midlife. Sharing experiences in a relaxed group setting can lessen the feeling of being alone in emotional shifts. Online forums can offer 24-hour support, though it is wise to be cautious about advice from unverified sources. Focus on supportive, respectful groups that do not push extreme solutions.

# Handling Low Mood Over the Long Term

### 1. Keep Expectations Realistic

Menopause can take years to transition completely. Mood changes may ease over time as hormones settle into post-menopausal patterns. It is helpful to remember that emotional changes do not always follow a neat schedule—there may be good weeks and harder ones.

### 2. Monitor Progress

If you try a new approach—like a short daily meditation or an herbal supplement (with a doctor's approval)—monitor how you feel over several weeks. Emotional improvements can be subtle at first. You might realize after a month that you are sleeping better or reacting with less annoyance to minor troubles.

### 3. Celebrate Small Gains

When you notice you handled a tricky situation more calmly than usual, acknowledge that progress. Even a small step like declining an invitation when you feel too overwhelmed is a way of self-care.

### 4. Stay Flexible

What worked at the start of menopause might need adjusting later on. Maybe at first, you found daily walks worked wonders, but later you needed to add a regular yoga-like stretch session or talk therapy to keep emotions balanced.

---

# Cultural and Social Factors

In some cultures, menopause is rarely discussed openly, leading women to feel shame or isolation about emotional swings. In others, older women are respected for their life experience, so menopause is viewed more neutrally. Recognize how your background might shape your comfort level discussing mood changes. Seeking out media, articles, or groups that speak to your cultural experience can help you feel validated.

# Could It Be Something Else?

While hormone changes can cause mood swings, do not overlook other potential causes:

- **Thyroid Imbalance**: Thyroid problems may mimic certain menopausal mood signs. A simple blood test can rule this out.
- **Chronic Stress or Grief**: If you are caring for aging parents, facing major work changes, or dealing with family tension, these stressors can add to emotional ups and downs.
- **Sleep Disorders**: Restless legs or sleep apnea might also disturb rest. Correcting these could boost mood.
- **Nutrient Deficiencies**: Low levels of vitamin B12, iron, or folate can lead to low energy and down feelings. Blood tests can check these levels.

A thorough medical check can ensure you address any underlying issues that might amplify menopause-related emotional concerns.

---

# When Professional Care is Needed

If emotions start hurting relationships or interfering with daily tasks, it is time to seek help. A mental health professional can:

- **Offer Therapy**: Techniques like cognitive behavioral approaches, which help reframe negative thoughts into more balanced ones.
- **Suggest Group Programs**: Some clinics have groups tailored for midlife women dealing with mood swings.
- **Provide Resources**: They may connect you with social workers, nutrition experts, or stress management classes.

Early support can prevent emotional concerns from turning into more complex problems.

---

# Talking to Family About Mood Changes

Even close relatives may not understand that menopause can involve emotional shifts. Clear communication reduces misunderstandings:

1. **Pick a Calm Moment**: Talk when you are not in the middle of a heated moment.
2. **Explain Physical Links**: A brief mention that hormone drops or poor sleep can affect mood might help them see this is not simply "overreacting."
3. **Ask for Specific Support**: If you want them to give you space when you first arrive home or to let you vent without judging, say so. Family members often want to help but might not know how.

## Balancing Work and Emotions

For women employed during menopause, mood issues can spill over into the workplace. Quick irritability or trouble focusing can harm productivity or lead to conflicts. Some tips:

- **Short Breaks**: If you sense frustration rising, excuse yourself for a quick walk or deep breaths.
- **Plan Tasks Wisely**: If mornings bring more energy, tackle tough tasks then.
- **Talk with HR**: If menopause is impacting your work significantly, some workplaces offer flexible schedules or can make small changes for comfort.
- **Stay Organized**: Writing a to-do list at the start of the day helps if your focus drifts. Cross off items as you finish them for a sense of control and progress.

## The Role of Laughter and Joy

Finding moments of humor or lightheartedness can ease tension. Watching a funny show, sharing jokes with a friend, or playing with a pet can lift a low mood. This does not mean ignoring real concerns, but it reminds you that joy and laughter are powerful tools for emotional health. Even in tough times, small pleasant moments can help counterbalance stress.

## Positive Self-Talk

Be mindful of how you speak to yourself internally. If you make a small mistake, you might feel the urge to say, "I'm so useless" or "I can't do anything right." Replacing this thought with something more balanced, like "I made a mistake, but I can fix it or learn from it," supports a gentler self-view. This shift can gradually reduce negative emotions linked with menopause.

## Summing Up Emotional Care

Menopause often brings mood shifts driven by hormonal changes, sleep issues, and life stress. You can manage these challenges through daily routines, healthy eating, movement, and stress reduction methods. Open communication with loved ones and checking in with health professionals can further support mood stability. For serious or long-lasting concerns, mental health experts can provide therapy or medication if needed. Remember that mood changes do not define who you are. With patience and the right actions, you can find steadier emotional footing during this life stage.

## Chapter 17 Conclusion

Emotional changes during menopause can be unsettling, but they make sense in the context of shifting hormones, nighttime rest problems, and daily life pressures. Many strategies—from breathing exercises to gentle movement—help regulate mood. Knowing when to seek professional help is also vital, as some women experience deeper low moods or anxious feelings that need more specialized care. Recognize that you are not alone, and many have navigated similar emotional shifts. By leaning on supportive relationships, sticking to healthy habits, and possibly working with a counselor or doctor, you can manage or even lessen many of the emotional hurdles that menopause can bring.

# Chapter 18: Handling Stress at Home and Work

Life events and obligations do not pause simply because you are going through menopause. In fact, this stage can coincide with raising teenagers, caring for aging parents, or juggling an intense job, all of which can compound stress. Hormonal changes may add irritability, poor sleep, or mental fatigue to the list of daily challenges. Managing stress effectively is key to staying emotionally steady and physically healthy.

This chapter explains why stress might feel stronger during menopause, shows how stress impacts the body and mind, and shares tips for reducing or managing it at home and in the workplace. We will look at different activities, organizational strategies, and communication styles that can help you respond to demands more calmly. By the end, you will have a clearer path to lowering the impact of stress, allowing you to navigate midlife changes with greater ease.

---

## Why Stress Feels Magnified in Midlife

### Hormonal Fluctuations

Estrogen and other hormones can influence how the brain handles pressure. When levels drop rapidly, the body's stress response can go into overdrive, making even small problems seem overwhelming. Physical signs like hot flashes or restlessness at night might further drain your tolerance for stress during the day.

### Multiple Responsibilities

Many women in midlife find themselves "sandwiched" between caring for older relatives while still supporting children or handling busy careers. Time and energy are limited resources. Add in everyday chores and finances, and it is no surprise that stress can escalate.

## Personal Transitions

Menopause can trigger deep thoughts about aging, body changes, or future plans. If you or your partner is also facing job changes or health shifts, that stress can pile up. Sometimes, a woman feels uncertain about identity or purpose after children leave home. All these factors can weigh on mental well-being.

---

# Identifying Signs of High Stress

1. **Tension Headaches** or muscle pains that do not seem connected to physical activity.
2. **Frequent Mood Swings** or a shorter fuse for anger or frustration.
3. **Trouble Sleeping**—stress can feed into insomnia or cause frequent waking.
4. **Digestive Problems**—upset stomach, changes in bowel habits, or recurring heartburn.
5. **Rapid Heartbeat** or a feeling of being on edge.
6. **Ongoing Fatigue** despite normal rest.

If these signs persist, it is a clue that your stress load might be too high. Taking steps to reduce or handle stress is crucial to avoid more serious health concerns like high blood pressure or major depression.

---

# Stress Management Basics

### 1. Recognize Triggers

Whether it is a difficult coworker, a crowded schedule, or an emotionally charged family event, pinpointing triggers helps you prepare solutions in advance. Some triggers might be avoidable, while others might need a plan to manage them effectively.

## 2. Physical Outlet

Movement helps release tension. A quick walk around the block when you feel overwhelmed can clear the mind. Simple chair exercises or stretches can also loosen tight muscles caused by stress. If you enjoy group classes, consider yoga-like or water aerobics sessions that incorporate mild forms of relaxation.

## 3. Mental Breaks

Small mental pauses throughout the day can keep stress from building up:

- **Mini-Breathing Sessions**: Close your eyes for 30 seconds, inhaling deeply and exhaling slowly.
- **Change of Scenery**: Step outside for a minute or two if possible, or look out a window to refocus.
- **Calm Music**: Keep a short playlist of soothing tunes to play when you need a quick de-stress.

## 4. Time Management

Organizing tasks and setting realistic deadlines can reduce last-minute chaos. If you often feel behind, consider using a planner or a digital calendar. Break large tasks into smaller steps, checking them off as you go, which offers a sense of control.

## 5. Self-Compassion

When hormones and life events create chaos, it is easy to be self-critical. Remind yourself that it is normal to feel overwhelmed. Speak kindly to yourself, the same way you might encourage a friend who is going through a tough time.

---

# Stress at Home: Strategies for Peace

## 1. Delegate Tasks

If you share a household with a partner, children, or other relatives, divide tasks. Many women feel they must handle cooking, cleaning, laundry, and errands solo. Instead, make a list of what needs doing and ask family members to pick tasks they can manage. This not only lightens your load but can teach responsibility to younger members of the family.

## 2. Simplify Meals

Cooking a large dinner after a busy day might be exhausting. Aim for simpler meals during the workweek—soups, stir-fries, or salads—and save more elaborate cooking for weekends or special occasions. A slow cooker or pressure cooker can help prepare balanced dishes with minimal time standing in the kitchen.

## 3. Set Boundaries

If extended family expects you to host big gatherings often, but you do not have the energy, it is okay to say no or propose a simpler plan. Constantly accommodating everyone else's preferences can push your stress level higher. Politely communicate your limits, like scheduling shorter visits or asking guests to bring dishes.

## 4. Find Your Calm Space

Having a quiet spot in the home—like a chair by a window or a corner with soft lighting—gives you a refuge when stress spikes. Even stepping away for five minutes can reset the mind. Let household members know you need a brief break and that it is not personal—it is for your sanity.

## 5. Shared Communication

Talk openly about menopause-related changes with family members if you feel comfortable. Explaining that hormonal shifts can intensify stress might reduce misunderstandings if you are more irritable or exhausted than normal.

---

# Stress at Work: Managing Job Pressures

Many women spend a large chunk of time at work, so reducing tension there is essential. Here are some approaches:

## 1. Organize Your Workspace

A clean, ordered workspace can ease the mind. Keep frequently used items within reach, and label or store documents properly to avoid frantic searching. If needed, spend a few minutes at the end of each day tidying up, so you start fresh the next morning.

## 2. Prioritize Tasks

When you arrive at work, list the tasks that need to be done, ordered by importance. If possible, tackle the most pressing or complex one first, when your mental energy is higher. This can prevent the dread of leaving big tasks until the last minute.

## 3. Time Blocking

Try scheduling blocks of time for email, phone calls, or specific projects rather than constantly switching tasks. Multitasking can increase mental strain. During a time block, focus on one set of tasks, then move on.

## 4. Speak Up about Needs

If menopause signs like hot flashes or low energy are making your work environment uncomfortable, see if small changes can help—like a desk fan, flexible break times, or adjusting the thermostat. A chat with a supervisor or HR might be beneficial. Some workplaces are open to adjusting conditions if it improves employee well-being.

## 5. Manage Interruptions

Constant interruptions can raise stress. If you get bombarded by colleagues or phone calls, consider using simple signals (like wearing headphones or setting an online status to "busy") during blocks of deep work. If certain colleagues frequently interrupt, politely ask if you can schedule a set time to talk so your workflow stays on track.

# Handling Stressful Interactions

## 1. Calm Communication

When faced with a tense conversation—at home or work—try not to respond immediately if you are upset. Take a breath, gather your thoughts, and speak more slowly. Explain your viewpoint plainly without accusing the other person. For example, say "I feel pressured when this happens," rather than "You always make things worse."

## 2. Problem-Solving Together

If a recurring issue is causing stress—like an ongoing disagreement with a coworker or repeated tension about household chores—suggest a collaborative approach. Ask, "What do you think would help both of us in this situation?" People often appreciate being invited to find a mutually beneficial solution.

## 3. Walk Away if Needed

In heated moments, stepping out of the conversation for a short break can keep emotions from boiling over. Say, "I need a quick moment to think. Let's talk again in ten minutes," then return once you have cooled down.

---

# Relaxation Techniques

## 1. Progressive Muscle Tensing

Sit or lie down. Tighten one muscle group, such as your feet, hold for a few seconds, then release. Move upward—legs, abdomen, arms, shoulders, face—tightening and releasing. This method helps pinpoint where stress is held in your body.

## 2. Visualization

Close your eyes and imagine a peaceful scene—a quiet beach, a calm lake, or a gentle forest. Picture all the details: sounds, smells, temperature. This mental break can briefly transport your mind away from stress. Even a minute or two can help refocus you.

### 3. Gentle Rhythmic Movement

Rocking in a rocking chair, swaying gently to quiet music, or even pacing slowly can calm the nervous system. This might sound simple, but repetitive motion can settle the body's stress response.

### 4. Warm Bath or Foot Soak

Heat relaxes muscles. Ending the day with a warm bath, or even just soaking your feet in warm water with a bit of Epsom salt, can melt tension away. If dryness or sensitivity is an issue, choose mild products without heavy fragrances.

---

## Technology and Stress

Digital devices can either help or add to stress:

- **Helpful Apps**: Some apps guide brief breathing exercises, relaxation tracks, or time management systems that lower disorganization.
- **Overstimulation**: Constant notifications, social media comparisons, or negative news can boost stress. It might help to turn off some alerts or set phone-free periods each day.
- **Online Communities**: Balanced, supportive online groups (for example, a midlife women's forum) can share coping ideas. But be cautious about excessive "doom-scrolling" or engaging in heated debates that raise stress.

---

## Social Support

Human connections are crucial for stress relief:

- **Friends and Peers**: Having someone to laugh with or talk over daily problems can cut tension. A short chat can sometimes reset your entire perspective.
- **Mentors**: In a work setting, a senior colleague can offer advice on dealing with workplace hurdles.
- **Support Groups**: Some women find comfort among others experiencing similar life changes. You might learn fresh stress-busting ideas from hearing others' stories.

---

# Mindset Shifts

### 1. Focus on What You Can Control

Often, stress grows when we worry about things we cannot change. Accepting that you cannot fix every problem can free mental space. Put energy into tasks or choices you can influence, and let go of the rest.

### 2. Adjust Expectations

If you have always been a perfectionist, midlife changes and added responsibilities might make that standard hard to maintain. This can fuel frustration. Aim for reasonable outcomes. Praise yourself for partial successes rather than dwelling on flaws.

### 3. Look for Positive Moments

Even on stressful days, there may be small spots of calm or laughter—a nice meal, a coworker's kind remark, or a moment with a pet. Recognizing these small positives can keep you from feeling like the entire day is ruined by stress.

---

# Handling Major Life Stressors

Sometimes stress is unavoidable due to serious events like a loved one's illness, job loss, or family crises. In those times:

1. **Seek Extra Support**: Lean on relatives, friends, or professionals. You might see a counselor or social worker to help navigate complex emotions and tasks.
2. **Set Priorities**: When under heavy strain, simplify. Cut non-essential activities. Focus on core tasks—health, critical family responsibilities, and key job duties.
3. **Stress-Release Routines**: Keep up simple daily habits like a warm shower or a few minutes of reading before bed. Routine helps build a sense of stability amid chaos.

## Physical Health Ties to Stress

Chronic stress can lead to:

- **Higher Blood Pressure**: Over time, constant strain can damage heart health.
- **Weak Immune Response**: You might catch colds more easily.
- **Increased Muscle Tension**: Leading to frequent aches or even tension headaches.
- **Weight Changes**: Some women eat more or less under stress, possibly leading to weight gain or other nutritional issues.

Balancing stress levels can help keep these health problems at bay. Pairing stress management with healthy eating, moderate exercise, and regular checkups can boost your overall resilience.

## Balancing Stress and Self-Care

### 1. Schedule Personal Time

It might feel odd to write "30 minutes of reading" on your calendar, but if that is what it takes to ensure you get time for yourself, do it. Let family or coworkers know that this slot is important for your well-being.

### 2. Avoid Over-Extending Yourself

If your schedule is jam-packed with appointments, volunteer tasks, social events, and work demands, it may be time to say no to new commitments. Practice polite but firm ways to decline, such as, "I'd love to, but my plate is full right now."

### 3. Practice Simple Gratitude

At the day's end, jot down one or two things that went right. These can be small—like enjoying a nice cup of tea or finishing a project on time. Focusing on what went well can balance out daily stresses.

## Workplace Flexibility

If menopause is causing noticeable problems, some workplaces offer certain flexibilities:

- **Remote or Hybrid Work**: If tasks allow, working from home part-time might reduce commute stress and help you manage hot flashes or schedule breaks.
- **Modified Hours**: Starting earlier or later could help if your energy pattern changes or if morning hot flashes are severe.
- **Ergonomic Adjustments**: A better chair, adjustable desk, or footrest can lower physical strain that adds to stress.

Asking about these options can feel intimidating, but a calm, clear discussion with HR or your supervisor may yield solutions.

## The Role of Counseling in Stress Reduction

A professional counselor can help you develop personalized strategies for stress. They might teach:

- **Cognitive Approaches**: Identifying unhelpful thought patterns that increase stress, and replacing them with more balanced thoughts.
- **Goal-Setting**: Breaking large problems into smaller, manageable actions.

- **Communication Skills**: Learning to speak your needs assertively at home or work.

Even a few sessions can equip you with new tools that support calmer living.

## Emotional Resilience

Stress does not vanish once menopause ends. Building emotional resilience is a lifelong skill. Steps like acknowledging your feelings, practicing self-care, and finding constructive outlets for tension can stay useful well beyond midlife. Women who become adept at managing stress often find they handle other life events with more stability, too.

## Setting Up a "Stress Toolkit"

Consider putting together a small set of go-to actions that help you calm down or refocus, for example:

- **Breathe**: A short breathing exercise.
- **Move**: Step outside or walk a flight of stairs.
- **Sip**: Drink water or a soothing tea.
- **Focus**: Write down tasks or feelings in a quick list.
- **Affirm**: A simple phrase that reminds you of your strength or of a hopeful viewpoint.

Keep this list on your phone or a small card. Practice these steps frequently so they become natural responses when stress flares.

## Summarizing Techniques

1. **Identify**: Know your top stress triggers—be it clutter, deadlines, or personal conflicts.

2. **Plan**: Have a strategy or step to address each trigger (e.g., schedule decluttering sessions, break down big deadlines, or use conflict resolution at home).
3. **Act**: Regularly apply these steps. Make time management a habit.
4. **Reflect**: Check what works and what does not. Adjust as needed.
5. **Remember Self-Care**: Nurturing your body and mind is not selfish; it is necessary for functioning well in everyday life.

# Chapter 18 Conclusion

Menopause can bring physical discomforts that amplify stress, especially when life is already busy with family duties or job tasks. Recognizing stress signals and learning to respond calmly helps you stay healthier and more balanced. Simple moves like decluttering your schedule, delegating tasks at home, and using brief relaxation techniques can reduce the toll stress takes on your mind and body. Communication skills—at home and work—are also key, since sharing your needs or limits can prevent misunderstandings.

Everyone's stress triggers differ, so try various approaches to discover what works best for you. With consistent effort, many women find that stress becomes more manageable. This leaves room for better focus on self-care, relationships, and personal growth—factors that can make the midlife years more positive and fulfilling. In the next chapters, we will continue looking at long-term health considerations and practical daily steps that support a better quality of life through and after menopause.

# Chapter 19: Staying Healthy in the Long Term

Menopause marks a significant milestone in a woman's life. But it does not mean growth or development ends. In fact, after menopause, many women continue to learn new skills, adapt to changing body needs, and build routines that support ongoing well-being. While previous chapters have covered specific concerns like hot flashes, dryness, or mood changes, this chapter takes a broader look at long-term health.

We will focus on how to maintain strength, mental clarity, and overall wellness in the years after menopause. We will cover medical checkups you might need, daily habits that can keep common issues at bay, and ways to adjust to your body's changing needs. By the end of this chapter, you should have a clear idea of how to build a plan that supports a healthy, active life for years ahead.

---

## Understanding Post-Menopause

Once menopause has passed—meaning a full year without menstrual cycles—a woman is considered in post-menopause. Hormone levels settle at lower levels, and you may find some signs of menopause (like hot flashes) begin to lessen over time. Other health matters, such as bone density and heart health, might require more attention. Each woman's experience is different, but awareness of potential risks can lead to better choices and fewer surprises.

### Common Changes in Post-Menopause

1. **Bone Density**: Bone thinning typically speeds up around menopause, then slows, but does not stop. Without proper care, bones might become weaker over time.
2. **Heart Concerns**: Low estrogen may slightly raise the chance of certain heart or blood vessel problems. Lifestyle habits can offset some of these risks.
3. **Body Composition**: Many women notice more weight around the midsection. Muscle mass may drop unless steps are taken to maintain it.

4. **Skin and Hair**: Lower levels of certain hormones can mean drier skin, hair thinning, or changes in texture.
5. **Bladder and Pelvic Floor**: Weaker pelvic support might lead to leaks when sneezing or laughing, known as stress incontinence.

Recognizing these general tendencies can help you plan ahead, whether that means getting regular checkups, exercising certain muscle groups, or adjusting your daily habits in ways that ease these changes.

---

# Regular Medical Checkups and Screenings

While you might no longer need visits related to menstrual cycles or childbirth, other checkups become more significant. Below are some appointments to consider scheduling:

## 1. Annual Physical Examination

A general checkup each year can catch issues early. Your doctor may measure blood pressure, check cholesterol levels, and ask about your activity and diet. Sometimes these visits include blood tests that show if anything (like blood sugar or thyroid function) is out of normal range.

## 2. Bone Density Scans

If you are in post-menopause, your doctor may suggest a DEXA scan to see how dense your bones are. This test is non-invasive and helps detect bone weakness early. If the results show thinning, the doctor can offer treatments or recommend changes in exercise, diet, or supplements (like calcium and vitamin D).

## 3. Heart Health Evaluations

Because heart risks can increase after menopause, it is wise to monitor this area regularly. This might involve:

- **Cholesterol Checks**: Ensuring LDL ("bad" cholesterol) and HDL ("good" cholesterol) levels are balanced.

- **Blood Pressure**: High readings can creep up without noticeable signs. Keeping it in normal ranges lowers strain on the heart.
- **Blood Sugar**: Checking for prediabetes or diabetes, since midlife weight shifts can affect glucose control.

## 4. Cancer Screenings

Talk with your doctor about the following:

- **Mammograms**: Most doctors advise regular mammograms based on age and risk factors.
- **Colon Checks**: Colonoscopy or other methods to look for signs of colon cancer are often recommended starting around age 45 to 50, and repeated as advised.
- **Cervical Checks**: Some guidelines suggest fewer Pap tests post-menopause, but that depends on past results and health history.

## 5. Eye and Dental Visits

Changes in hormone levels can affect vision or gum health. Regular dental cleanings help prevent gum problems, and an eye exam can catch issues like glaucoma or dryness that some women face.

---

# Diet for Long-Term Wellness

Eating patterns can affect how you feel both physically and mentally as you age. Certain nutrients become even more important after menopause:

## 1. Calcium and Vitamin D

These two are vital for bones. Calcium supports bone structure, while vitamin D aids calcium absorption. Good sources include:

- **Dairy Products**: Milk, cheese, and yogurt (if tolerated).
- **Fortified Plant Milks**: Check labels for added calcium and vitamin D if you avoid dairy.
- **Leafy Greens**: Spinach, kale, and collard greens.

- **Sun Exposure**: In moderation, to help the body produce vitamin D naturally.

## 2. Protein

Maintaining muscle mass can become more challenging post-menopause. Lean protein sources include chicken, fish, beans, nuts, or low-fat dairy. Try to have some protein with each meal—perhaps an egg or beans at breakfast, chicken or tofu at lunch, and fish or lentils at dinner.

## 3. Fiber and Antioxidants

Fiber helps keep the digestive system moving and can support healthy cholesterol and blood sugar levels. Fruits, veggies, beans, and whole grains are good sources. Antioxidant-rich foods (berries, leafy greens, carrots) may help lower oxidative stress in the body. They are not a magic cure for everything, but they can support overall health.

## 4. Healthy Fats

Focus on fats from sources like avocados, nuts, seeds, and olive oil. These can help with heart health. Avoid too many saturated fats (like those in butter or certain cuts of red meat) or trans fats found in some packaged baked goods.

## 5. Hydration

Post-menopause dryness can show up in the skin, eyes, or even private areas. Drinking enough water helps maintain fluid balance. If plain water feels boring, add cucumber slices, a bit of fruit juice, or herbal teas for flavor.

---

# Physical Activity for Strength and Flexibility

Many post-menopausal women worry about losing muscle or noticing more stiffness in joints. Regular movement addresses these concerns:

## 1. Resistance Exercises

These can be done with small weights, resistance bands, or even bodyweight moves (like squats, modified push-ups, and lunges). Building or keeping muscle can help with balance, posture, and the ability to do daily tasks without getting hurt.

## 2. Weight-Bearing Cardio

Activities like walking, dancing, or light jogging put mild stress on bones, which signals them to stay strong. Even 30 minutes a few times a week can make a difference. If high-impact exercise is too hard on your joints, brisk walking or low-impact aerobics can still be beneficial.

## 3. Stretching and Balance

Gentle stretches improve range of motion and help prevent stiffness. Balance moves, like standing on one foot briefly (while holding a stable chair for safety), can lower the risk of falls. Some people explore practices like tai chi or certain yoga-like routines to blend balance, stretching, and calm breathing.

## 4. Respecting Limitations

If you have joint problems or other constraints, talk to a doctor or physical therapist about modified exercises. Even small sessions add up. Consistency matters more than doing intense workouts once in a while.

---

# Protecting Cognitive Function

Maintaining clear thinking and memory is a goal for many as they age. While serious memory issues can have many causes, certain habits support brain health:

1. **Ongoing Learning**: Challenge your mind by trying new activities, whether it is learning a language, playing puzzles, or taking an online course.
2. **Social Connections**: Interacting with friends or community groups keeps the mind active and can lower feelings of isolation.

3. **Physical Exercise**: Regular movement supports blood flow to the brain and can help preserve clarity.
4. **Adequate Rest**: Good sleep helps the brain consolidate memories and repair itself. Trouble sleeping is common post-menopause, so see earlier chapters for strategies to improve rest.
5. **Healthy Diet**: Nutrients that help the heart typically help the brain as well. Omega-3 fats (from fish or certain nuts) may play a role in supporting normal brain function.

## Emotional Wellness Over the Years

Menopause can bring emotional swings, but post-menopause also has its emotional demands, from adjusting to an empty nest to dealing with aging parents or grandparent roles. Some helpful steps:

- **Stay Connected**: Regular calls, visits, or online chats with loved ones can keep you feeling part of a community.
- **Seek Purposeful Activities**: Volunteer work, hobbies, or mentoring younger people can bring a sense of fulfillment.
- **Handle Stress**: Develop routines that reduce tension, like a short breathing practice or a 10-minute stroll outside each morning.
- **Know Your Boundaries**: If family or community expectations overload you, learn to say "I can't take that on right now."

## Sexual Health in the Long Run

Even if dryness or other concerns caused discomfort before, many women remain active in this area well past menopause. If dryness persists, lubricants or local estrogen (discussed in earlier chapters) can help. Communication with a partner is key. If interest changes, or if other physical factors come into play (like aches or energy levels), speaking openly can lead to adjustments that keep closeness enjoyable.

# Keeping Track of Your Own Health Numbers

It is helpful to learn and monitor certain health markers so you can spot changes early and adjust accordingly. Some key measures:

1. **Blood Pressure**: High numbers may indicate more strain on the heart.
2. **Cholesterol Levels**: Keep total cholesterol, LDL, HDL, and triglycerides in healthy ranges.
3. **Blood Sugar or A1C**: Helps detect early signs of impaired glucose control.
4. **Body Weight or Waist Circumference**: Rapid gains around the midsection might suggest an issue with diet or hormones that you can address.
5. **Bone Density**: If you have a baseline test, you can compare future scans to see if you are losing bone mass.

Keep records of these results and bring them to doctor visits. Trends over time can show whether changes in diet, exercise, or medication are making a difference.

---

# Financial Planning for Health Needs

As you move past menopause, considering future health costs can lower stress. Some points to think about:

- **Insurance Coverage**: If available, understand what your plan covers in terms of screenings or procedures.
- **Emergency Funds**: Setting aside a small "health savings" cushion can help if unexpected medical bills pop up.
- **Flexible Spending or Health Savings Accounts**: If your employer offers these, contributing to them might save money for medical-related expenses.
- **Long-Term Care**: Though not everyone needs extended care, it is wise to learn about possible costs and options for later years.

# Adjusting to Body Changes Kindly

Weight gain around the waist or slower metabolism can test your self-confidence. A few reminders:

1. **Focus on Health Indicators**: Instead of fixating on a certain size, watch how your clothes fit, your energy levels, and your test results.
2. **Avoid Extreme Diets**: Sudden, harsh restrictions are hard to keep up and can harm muscle or bone health. Focus on balanced approaches that you can maintain for the long term.
3. **Celebrate Strength**: Muscle is key to independent living. If you see progress in lifting a heavier grocery bag or climbing stairs with less effort, that is a win.
4. **Wear Comfortable Clothes**: Outfits that fit well can boost daily confidence. Let go of items that make you feel squeezed or self-conscious.

---

# Social and Community Involvement

Staying engaged with the world around you can bring a sense of connection and purpose. Examples:

- **Clubs or Groups**: Book clubs, walking clubs, or community sports leagues may welcome participants of all ages.
- **Volunteering**: Schools, libraries, hospitals, or local charities often need extra hands. This can be a meaningful way to pass on your experience.
- **Senior Centers**: Some have fitness classes, social lunches, and other events suited to a range of ages.
- **Online Communities**: If you prefer to stay at home or have mobility concerns, online groups can offer social interaction, though try to balance screen time with offline activities, too.

---

# Supplements and Medicines

After menopause, some women use supplements to fill nutrient gaps. A few pointers:

- **Calcium and Vitamin D**: A common recommendation for women worried about bone health.
- **Omega-3s**: Found in fish oil or flaxseed supplements, may help with heart and brain function, though results vary.
- **Multivitamins**: Some choose a basic formula designed for age 50+ to cover general needs.
- **Prescription Drugs**: In certain cases, doctors may prescribe medicines for bone density, heart conditions, or other issues. Following the dosage and attending follow-up appointments is essential for safe results.

Always speak with a qualified health professional before starting any new supplement, as interactions or side effects can happen if you also take prescription medicines.

## Emotional Transitions and Identity

Post-menopause can be a phase of life redefinition. Children might have moved out, or you might be nearing retirement. While this can be liberating, it can also bring feelings of uncertainty. Handling these changes with thought can help:

- **Reflect on Goals**: Are there new hobbies or projects you have always wanted to start?
- **Seek Support**: A counselor or life coach can help you examine your options if you feel stuck.
- **Try New Roles**: Maybe you have an opportunity to mentor younger coworkers or volunteer with youth groups. Passing on your knowledge can be fulfilling.
- **Build Friendships**: Maintaining old friendships or forming new ones can keep you grounded. Social ties can help lower stress and keep you motivated.

## Sleep Quality After Menopause

While many find that severe night sweats may lessen over time, some still have trouble sleeping. A few reminders:

1. **Cool Bedroom**: Use a fan or air conditioning, and choose lightweight blankets.
2. **Avoid Large Meals at Night**: Indigestion can disrupt rest.
3. **Limit Late Caffeine**: Even mid-afternoon coffee might keep some people awake later.
4. **Tech-Free Wind-Down**: Put away phones or tablets an hour before bed, replacing them with a quiet activity like reading or mild stretches.

If sleep problems persist, consult a doctor. Persistent rest troubles can affect memory, mood, and physical health over time.

## Maintaining Independence

Many women aim to stay independent as they age. Key factors include:

- **Physical Strength**: Regular exercise for muscles and balance can minimize the risk of falls.
- **Medical Monitoring**: Catching issues early means less chance of them becoming major concerns.
- **Financial Preparedness**: Having resources to handle unexpected events supports independence.
- **Social Network**: Trusted friends or neighbors can help if sudden difficulties happen, like a minor health crisis.

Preparing for the unexpected does not mean living fearfully; it simply means having a plan in place so you can adapt without feeling helpless if a challenge arises.

## Taking Advantage of Free or Low-Cost Services

Many local communities, health centers, or nonprofits offer:

- **Nutrition Workshops**: Teaching meal prep or healthy cooking at no or low cost.
- **Exercise Programs**: Senior community centers or health clubs might have discounted memberships or classes.

- **Health Screenings**: Some organizations provide free blood pressure checks, cholesterol tests, or bone density scans at community events.
- **Counseling Hotlines**: For emotional support during tough times.

Check local bulletins, libraries, or government websites to find out what is available.

## Planning for Future Goals

Post-menopause can be a time to consider personal plans, whether it is learning a new skill, traveling (if finances and health allow), or moving to a different home. Laying out these intentions can bring a sense of enthusiasm:

1. **Short-Term Goals**: Maybe you want to start a vegetable garden this year or learn a craft.
2. **Medium-Term Goals**: In the next few years, you might plan a trip, update your home, or consider part-time work if you are semi-retired.
3. **Long-Term Goals**: Think about where you want to live later in life, how you want to spend your time, and how you will pay for it.

Sharing these thoughts with a partner or a friend can spark ideas and motivate you to take small steps toward them.

## Maintaining a Sense of Humor

Life after menopause has its share of challenges, but humor can smooth the edges. Laughing at minor mishaps—like forgetting why you walked into a room—can break tension. Spending time with positive, friendly people who enjoy a good laugh can keep you feeling upbeat. It does not mean ignoring serious concerns, but it helps place them in a balanced perspective.

## Final Thoughts on Long-Term Health

Menopause is not just an end; it is also a new phase where you can continue shaping your lifestyle for resilience and contentment. Consistent habits in eating, movement, and stress management can help you remain strong and active. Keeping track of key health markers, scheduling important checkups, and staying socially engaged all form part of a well-rounded plan.

Each woman's path is unique, and it is fine to adjust as you learn more about yourself. If something you tried a few years ago no longer suits you, change it. Stay curious, stay open to new experiences, and remember that health includes both body and mind. By paying attention to the hints your body gives and by seeking professional advice when needed, you can look forward to many vibrant years post-menopause.

## Chapter 19 Conclusion

Staying healthy in the long term after menopause involves paying attention to bones, heart, mood, and more. Regular medical visits and certain screenings become vital tools in catching issues early. Keeping a balanced diet with enough protein, calcium, and fiber is key, alongside consistent exercise that supports muscle and bone strength. Emotional well-being, cognitive function, and social connections also matter deeply. By tending to these different areas, you build a foundation that can help you remain active, alert, and in charge of your life.

In the next (and final) chapter, we will bring together many of the ideas covered in this book. You will find practical steps for daily life that combine good nutrition, smart movement, emotional balance, and more. With a clear and organized approach, you can craft routines that match your needs, stay flexible, and adjust to changes as you move through post-menopause with confidence.

# Chapter 20: Practical Steps for Daily Life

This final chapter gathers essential points from the entire book, wrapping them into a clear, step-by-step framework you can adapt to your routine. Menopause and the years that follow may bring changes to the body, emotions, and relationships, but with practical actions, you can handle many of these shifts in ways that fit your preferences and lifestyle.

We will look at creating daily schedules, handling stress quickly, organizing checkups, and forming a personal support network. Consider this chapter a set of tools you can choose from, picking what feels right for your unique situation. You might tailor it over time, swapping out techniques or adding new ones as your needs change. The goal is to move forward feeling stable, capable, and at peace with the changes menopause brings.

---

## Building a Day-to-Day Routine

### 1. Morning Start

- **Hydration**: Drinking a glass of water soon after waking helps the body wake up.
- **Gentle Movement**: A short stretch session can loosen stiff muscles. If you have more time, a brisk walk or mild exercise can get blood flowing.
- **Light Breakfast**: Focus on fiber, protein, and healthy fats—maybe oatmeal with nuts or an egg with whole grain toast.
- **Breathing Pause**: Even two minutes of slow, controlled breaths can reduce morning tension.

### 2. Midday Break

- **Check in with Yourself**: How do you feel physically or mentally? If you sense irritability or fatigue, do a quick stress reducer, like a short walk or calm breathing.

- **Balanced Lunch**: Try a mix of protein (chicken, tofu, or beans), whole grains (brown rice or quinoa), and vegetables. This combination supports stable blood sugar.
- **Hydrate Again**: Keep a water bottle nearby. Flavor it with lemon slices or cucumber if plain water is dull.

### 3. Late Afternoon Checkpoint

- **Mini Exercise Burst**: Stand up if you have been sitting a lot. Do a few squats, shoulder rolls, or a short walk around the block.
- **Snack Wisely**: Choose fruit, nuts, yogurt, or vegetable sticks to keep energy up. Avoid high sugar items that can lead to a crash later.
- **Plan for Evening**: Think about what you will have for dinner. If it is a busy night, maybe a quick soup or salad is easiest.

### 4. Evening Wind-Down

- **Light Dinner**: Aim for a balanced plate of vegetables, lean protein, and maybe a small serving of whole grains. Avoid eating large, heavy meals too close to bedtime.
- **Limit Caffeine**: Stop caffeine intake by mid-afternoon or earlier if you notice it disrupts rest.
- **Reduce Screen Time**: Give yourself an hour off phones, tablets, or laptops before sleeping if possible.
- **Relaxing Ritual**: A warm bath, mild foot soak, gentle stretching, or reading can signal the brain to start calming.

### 5. Bedtime Routine

- **Cool Environment**: Set the bedroom temperature a bit lower to address any potential night sweats.
- **Minimal Light**: Use curtains or shades to block external light. Soft lamps or night-lights help if you must get up but avoid bright lights.
- **Set a Regular Time**: Going to sleep and waking up at consistent times aids in restful nights.

# Weekly and Monthly Planning

## Weekly Habits

- **Meal Prep**: Carve out a bit of time (like Sunday afternoon) to wash and chop vegetables, cook a big batch of grains or soup, and plan the week's dinners.
- **Exercise Scheduling**: Write down your workout times—like two strength sessions, three walks—so you know what to expect.
- **Household Chores**: Spread them out instead of letting them pile up, or assign tasks to family members if possible.
- **Set a Goal**: Each week, choose a small health or stress-management goal—like drinking an extra glass of water each day or taking one new walk route.

## Monthly Tasks

- **Check Your Health Numbers**: If you have a blood pressure machine or can stop at a pharmacy with a free kiosk, note your reading. Track it to see trends.
- **Weigh-In or Waist Measurement**: While the scale is not everything, it can spot trends. If you see weight creeping up significantly, you can adjust your diet or movement.
- **Social Calendar**: Plan a fun outing with friends or family. Keep connections strong.
- **Review Finances**: If you are saving for health expenses or future goals, check your budget to ensure you are on track.

## Seasonal or Yearly Items

- **Medical Checkups**: Schedule bone density, mammograms, or blood tests as recommended.
- **Physical Challenges**: Maybe each season you aim to walk a local trail or join a group activity to keep your body active in new ways.
- **Declutter**: Clearing out old items from closets or the pantry can lower stress and keep your environment inviting.

# Quick Stress Handling Methods

1. **Breathing Set**: Inhale for four counts, hold for one, exhale for four counts. Repeat a few times.
2. **Grounding**: Look around and identify five objects you see, four you feel, three you hear, two you smell, and one you taste or sense. This brings the mind to the present.
3. **Body Scan**: Close your eyes and mentally scan from your toes up to your head, checking for tension. If you find a tight spot, pause to relax that area.
4. **Positive Phrase**: Repeat a brief saying like, "I can handle what comes next," or, "One step at a time."

---

# Adjusting for Menopause-Related Concerns

## Hot Flashes or Sweats

- **Layer Clothes**: So you can remove a sweater or jacket when you feel heat coming on.
- **Carry a Small Fan**: Handheld or battery-powered fans can offer quick relief in public.
- **Mind Your Meal Choices**: If spicy foods trigger warmth, limit them or eat them earlier in the day.

## Vaginal Dryness

- **Keep Lubricants Handy**: Over-the-counter lubricants or moisturizers can be discreetly stored in a bathroom drawer.
- **Stay Hydrated**: This can support overall tissue hydration.
- **Discuss Options**: If dryness is severe, local estrogen might be a solution. Consult your doctor.

## Mood Fluctuations

- **Schedule Breaks**: Plan mini mental rests if you know certain times of day are more stressful.

- **Communicate**: Let close friends or family know if you are feeling on edge, so they understand it is not personal.
- **Counseling**: If mood swings become intense, short-term talk therapy can be helpful.

## Sleep Difficulties

- **Evening Routine**: Consistency is key. Try to settle in for bed at the same time, using calming activities.
- **Watch Caffeine**: Cut back if you notice restlessness at night.
- **Room Setup**: Good pillows, supportive mattress, and the right temperature can make a big difference.

---

# Constructing Your Personal Support Network

No one is meant to handle everything alone. Building a team around you for emotional, practical, or health support is valuable.

### 1. Family and Friends

- **Spouse or Partner**: Let them know how they can help—maybe by cooking a meal on busy days or giving you a quiet hour to rest.
- **Close Friends**: They can be a sounding board for daily frustrations or share tips they have learned.
- **Children or Siblings**: Ask for help with errands or appointments if mobility or time is an issue.

### 2. Medical Professionals

- **Primary Doctor**: Your first resource for general questions, checkups, or referrals.
- **Women's Health Specialist**: May understand menopause-related signs in more depth.
- **Mental Health Expert**: Counseling can guide you through emotional dips, transitions, or relationship challenges.
- **Physical Therapist**: If you have pain or need specific exercises for better posture, balance, or strength.

3. **Community Groups**

   - **Meetups for Women in Midlife**: Sharing experiences, successes, or challenges can lighten the load.
   - **Local or Online Forums**: If you cannot find a group nearby, online communities can offer support. Be selective to ensure you join a positive, encouraging space.

---

## Practical Life Skills for Ongoing Vitality

1. **Learn Basic Home Repairs**: Feeling competent around the house can boost confidence and reduce stress if something minor breaks.
2. **Budgeting**: Understanding income and expenses, setting up basic savings, and planning for future medical needs lowers financial strain.
3. **Cooking Methods**: Master a few easy, healthy meals to avoid last-minute unhealthy takeout.
4. **Time Management**: A paper planner or phone calendar can keep you on track with appointments and activities, so you do not feel overwhelmed.

---

## Handling Shifts in Family Roles

As children grow up or parents age, your role might shift:

- **Adult Children**: They may move out or come back home for a while. Setting boundaries and mutual respect is key. You are still a parent, but they are more independent.
- **Grandchildren**: If you choose to help care for them, balance your own needs with the new responsibilities.
- **Aging Parents**: Caring for older relatives can be rewarding yet stressful. Seek help from siblings, community services, or respite care if needed.

## Ideas for Mental Stimulation

- **Puzzles and Games**: Crossword puzzles, sudoku, or word games can keep the mind sharp.
- **Reading**: Both fiction and nonfiction can expand thinking and give topics for discussion with friends.
- **Creative Hobbies**: Painting, writing, knitting, or crafting can offer a sense of achievement and calm.
- **Technology Lessons**: If you are not comfortable with computers or smartphones, local libraries or senior centers often have free or low-cost classes.

## Avoiding Isolation

Loneliness can creep in as life changes around you. Combat this by:

- **Scheduling Social Events**: Even a coffee date or video call each week with a friend can lift spirits.
- **Volunteering**: A chance to meet like-minded people while doing good for others.
- **Local Activities**: Check community calendars for fairs, concerts, or clubs that spark your interest.

## Healthy Ways to Celebrate Milestones

While we are avoiding certain words related to "celebration," it is still good to mark personal achievements or birthdays in a meaningful way:

- **Plan a Simple Gathering**: Invite a couple of friends or relatives for a cozy meal.
- **Write Down Accomplishments**: Note what you are proud of, like mastering a new recipe or improving your walking endurance.
- **Reflect**: Take a quiet half-hour to think about what you have done well over the past year and what you hope to do next.

## Keeping a Positive Outlook

Menopause can feel overwhelming at times, but focusing on constructive problem-solving and small acts of gratitude can build resilience:

- **Gratitude Notes**: Jot down two or three good things that happened each day, however minor.
- **View Challenges as Learnings**: If you have a tough day, reflect on what might help next time.
- **Surround Yourself with Positivity**: Music, photos, or shows that bring a smile can shift mood quickly when stress arises.

## Long-Term Planning for Comfort

1. **Assess Your Living Space**: Could your home be adapted easily as you age? Are there many stairs or hard-to-reach cabinets? Sometimes small changes, like grab bars in the bathroom, can provide peace of mind.
2. **Financial Safety**: Even minor savings each month can add up, giving you a cushion if unexpected costs show up.
3. **Emergency Contacts**: Keep important numbers—doctor, nearby relatives, a reliable neighbor—on your phone or a fridge magnet.
4. **Wills and Documents**: If you have not organized estate planning or medical directives, consider doing so. It simplifies decisions for everyone if an emergency arises.

## Putting It All Together: A Sample Plan

Below is an example of how a typical day might look, pulling together many of the tips we have discussed:

- **7:00 AM**: Wake up, drink a glass of water, do 10 minutes of gentle stretches or a short walk outside if weather allows.
- **7:30 AM**: Quick shower, then have a protein-rich breakfast (scrambled eggs with veggies, or yogurt with fruit and nuts). Review your to-do list for the day.

- **Mid-Morning**: If you are working, tackle your most demanding tasks first. Every hour, stand up and move for a minute or two to avoid stiffness.
- **12:30 PM**: Balanced lunch—salad with chicken or beans, whole grain roll, piece of fruit. If possible, take a 10-minute walk outside for fresh air.
- **2:00 PM**: If tiredness creeps in, do a quick breathing exercise or sip water. Keep healthy snacks like carrots, hummus, or nuts close by.
- **5:30 PM**: Prepare a simple dinner with fish or poultry, roasted vegetables, and maybe brown rice. If pressed for time, use items prepped on the weekend.
- **7:00 PM**: Leisure time—could be reading, calling a friend, or a mild hobby. Limit phone notifications to reduce digital clutter.
- **8:30 PM**: Begin winding down—dim lights, avoid caffeine, maybe take a warm bath or do 10 minutes of calm stretches.
- **9:30-10:00 PM**: Bedtime, ensuring the room is at a cooler temperature. Keep water near the bed in case of nighttime thirst.

This is just an illustration. Modify it for your schedule, energy level, and preferences.

## Maintaining Flexibility Over Time

No plan is static, especially during or after menopause. If you find that an exercise routine no longer suits your joints, switch to a more comfortable method, like water-based workouts. If a new medical condition arises, adapt your diet or checkup schedule accordingly. The key is to remain open to making adjustments as you learn what supports your body and mind best.

## Chapter 20 Conclusion

Practical steps for daily life during and after menopause can make a real difference in how you feel each day. By creating consistent routines—whether it is morning stretches, balanced meals, or a calm wind-down at night—you give your mind and body the steady support they need. Weekly and monthly planning keeps you on track with health checkups, chores, and social activities, preventing overwhelm. Remember to handle stress proactively through short breaks, deep breathing, or creative hobbies.

Keeping a personal support network of friends, family, and professionals ensures you have help and encouragement as you face ups and downs. Building a balanced approach to work, relationships, and personal time can maintain both energy and emotional stability. As you use these tips, feel free to adapt them to what feels right for you. Over the years, your needs may shift, but the core ideas—consistency, self-care, and staying informed—will continue to be valuable.

With this final chapter, you have a comprehensive guide to handling menopause and the years that follow. You have learned about physical health, emotional well-being, social connections, and practical daily steps. Apply what resonates with you, stay curious about new methods, and remember that each small effort adds up to a healthier, more comfortable life path. You deserve to move forward with assurance, equipped with an array of strategies that can lighten the load and boost your overall satisfaction in the years ahead.

www.ingramcontent.com/pod-product-compliance
Lightning Source LLC
LaVergne TN
LVHW012044070526
838202LV00056B/5590